Cooking Without

Note to the Reader

The recipes and information in this book are not meant to be prescriptive. Any attempt to treat a medical condition should always come under the direction of a competent physician. Neither the publishers nor the author can accept responsibility for illness arising from a failure by a reader to take medical advice.

Cooking
Without

*Recipes free from added gluten, sugar, dairy
products, yeast, salt and saturated fat*

BARBARA COUSINS

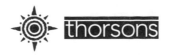

Thorsons

An Imprint of HarperCollinsPublishers

77–85 Fulham Palace Road

Hammersmith, London W6 8JB

The website address is: www.thorsonselement.com

First published by Barbara Cousins 1989

First published by Thorsons 1997

This edition 2000

11 13 15 14 12 10

Barbara Cousins 1997, 2000

Barbara Cousins asserts the moral right to

be identified as the author of this work

A catalogue record for this book

is available from the British Library

ISBN 0 7225 4022 1

Printed and bound in Great Britain by

Martins The Printers Ltd, Berwick upon Tweed

Contents

Foreword

Improving your health through diet can be daunting unless you have some help with creating appetizing menus. We all know what we shouldn't eat, but what do we do with those healthy ingredients like brown rice, vegetables and pulses? Few cookery books dwell on them for long, and those that do usually combine them with flour, butter or margarine, cheese, eggs and other dairy products. That's not much help for someone who is serious about trying to discover whether they have any food allergies.

Barbara Cousins is a working nutritional therapist, and her book has arisen out of the need to help many people find ways to really enjoy food cooked without all those ingredients we so often take for granted. I have not come across any other book which contains so many recipes using vegetables in appetizing ways. Now that the World Health Organization is advising all of us to eat at least five portions of fruit and vegetables every day, good recipes are vitally important, and you are sure to find some in *Cooking Without* that you will treasure and use over and over again.

Linda Lazarides

Introduction

This book is about health – how to gain it and how to keep it. Health is not a mere absence of disease, but a positive feeling of well-being which embraces mental, emotional and spiritual as well as physical health. This book is about the nutritional aspects of health, the dos and don'ts of healthy eating because, quite simply, we are what we eat. By giving the body a sufficient amount of the nutrients it needs, it has the best opportunity to heal itself and to stay well.

Detoxification

The two main causes of health problems are toxicity and malnutrition. In Western society, we are overfed but under nourished. If our bodies receive sufficient good quality fuel (in the form of vitamins and minerals) then they will be aided to work more efficiently and to overcome any toxicity (substances which should not be present in the body). Similarly, if we receive insufficient amounts of essential nutrients our toxic load may be allowed to rise to levels which promote ill health.

Where Does Toxicity Originate From?

In my opinion, the main sources of toxicity are as follows:

- Some toxicity in food is natural, such as solanine in potatoes. Most, however, is unnatural, such as fungicides, pesticides, colourings, flavourings and stabilizers.

- Industrial emissions, cigarette smoke and exhaust fumes pollute our atmosphere.
- Our drinking water is polluted by both industry and farming, as well as by the chemicals used to 'cleanse' it.
- Most drugs contain toxins, including over-the-counter remedies such as laxatives, painkillers and indigestion tablets. Alcohol is a poison.
- Around our homes, deodorant, perfume, skin care products, washing-up liquid and other cleansing fluids are chemically derived toxic substances, which are absorbed to a certain extent by our bodies.
- Bottled-up feelings and emotions constitute emotional toxicity which in turn affects our physical well being.

Toxicity and Ill Health

It is impossible for us to avoid toxins completely. Indeed, our bodies are built to cope with a certain amount, the liver being our main organ of detoxification. Toxins are naturally removed from our bodies through urine and faeces, sweating and expiration (breathing out). It is only when these elimination channels cannot cope with this removal that the body will let us know that all is not well by producing certain symptoms.

The safest place for excess toxins to overflow is through the skin, as this is farthest away from the vital internal organs and enables toxicity to be removed to the outside world. The boils and carbuncles so common in the past were the result of toxins being eliminated through the skin. Nowadays, these are less common. Even those teenagers who live on chocolate and chips frequently have good complexions. It takes a certain amount of vitality for the body to be able to eliminate excess toxins through the skin, and many individuals do not have constitutions strong enough for this process. Health problems such as psoriasis, eczema, rashes, itching, dandruff, boils and spots are caused by this elimination process.

Even if the body does not have the vitality to use the skin successfully to eliminate excess toxins, it does not give up trying. The next safest place for it to use is the internal mucosa; that is any moist orifices open to the outside world. Eliminating in this way causes illnesses such as coughs, colds, catarrh, diarrhoea, colitis, thrush, cystitis, conjunctivitis, ulcers and heavy, clotted periods.

Individuals who still have excess toxicity, even though their bodies may be using some of the above methods to eliminate toxins, will suffer from symptoms related to toxicity being deposited in the body, usually in the areas of least resistance. These areas vary from person to person, and are dependent on factors such as hereditary conditions, illnesses and injuries. Tiredness, irritability, anxiety, depression, arthritis, high blood pressure, heart problems and cancer are just some of the problems which can be promoted by toxicity.

Needless to say, everyone can benefit from a period of detoxification, whether they have serious health problems, just feel below par or are healthy and want to make sure that they stay that way.

The Health Benefits of Cooking Without

Following the eating regime outlined in this book will reduce the toxic load and improve the level of nutrients available to the body. Also, because the diet is easy for the body to assimilate, the food travels quickly through the digestive tract. This not only assists the removal of toxins, but because the body's workload is reduced, it also releases extra energy for healing and elimination. Additionally, the diet is designed to support the body's blood sugar, and by doing so, not only does the individual feel better but every organ and system in the body feels healthier and works more efficiently, too.

Some Common Health Problems

Low Blood Sugar (Hypoglycaemia)

We need sugar in order to fuel our bodies and our brains, but it needs to be in the right form. The sugar we find in biscuits and sweets and add to our tea is not a good fuel. This sugar has been over processed and is too readily absorbed by the body. It causes a sudden surge of sugar to enter the bloodstream. Because too much sugar in the bloodstream is harmful, the pancreas must produce extra insulin to remove this excess. In order to do this, the pancreas needs fuel and energy, and so eating sugar robs our body of vital nutrients and overworks the pancreas.

If, however, we eat sugar in the form of complex carbohydrate foods (such as rice, millet and root vegetables) then the body slowly breaks these down into simple sugars (glucose) which are steadily released into the bloodstream to give us sustained energy. If we eat more at a particular meal than the body needs, then the excess glucose is converted into glycogen and stored by the liver so that, mid-morning or mid-afternoon, we can have a top-up of blood sugar.

Unfortunately, not everyone's liver is giving them a good blood sugar releasing service. This is usually because the liver is struggling to cope with excess toxins and a lack of nutrients. As far as the body is concerned, removal of excess toxins is more important than giving the body or brain energy, and there is a tendency for the liver to say, 'Sit down if you are tired or cannot think straight – I've got too much to do!' Hence, many individuals develop cravings for sugary snacks in order to boost their blood sugar, and the vicious circle starts again. Tea, coffee and cigarettes also boost blood sugar – they do this by kicking the adrenal glands into action.

Living on the adrenal glands is an alternative way to produce energy as this causes blood sugar to be released from cells. However, adrenalin is designed for emergency situations – the 'flight or fight' response – and is not meant to be experienced daily. Nowadays, many individuals have adrenal glands which are becoming exhausted due to overuse. At one end of the scale are individuals who feel tired and always seem to be pushing themselves to keep going, and at the other end we have those suffering from illnesses such as Chronic Fatigue Syndrome (ME), see page 17. In between is a list of symptoms related to low blood sugar (hypoglycaemia), and these can affect not only the physical body but also the mental and emotional states. They include fatigue, headaches, palpitations, weak or dizzy spells, cold sweats, cravings, unjustified fears, lack of concentration or a muzzy head, mental confusion, depression, anxiety, phobias, restlessness, moodiness, insomnia, night terrors, uncoordination and a lack of or excessive appetite. Low blood sugar also underlies most other health problems.

By putting *Cooking Without* into practice, foods eaten at regular intervals are used to keep the blood sugar stable, thereby allowing the liver and adrenal glands to recover and the body to obtain sufficient energy to remove excess toxins. When the blood sugar is more stable you will be aware that your mood and your energy are more even and that you do not develop cravings. Other symptoms related to low blood sugar will also disappear.

When trying to improve health it is important to be aware that our bodies can only produce a certain amount of energy each day, and that this energy is needed for detoxification and healing. For instance, if you feel a little better and decide to catch up on all those jobs you have left undone, then you may start to feel poorly again because the energy has started going into the jobs rather than into healing. It is therefore important to allow a period of convalescence, when you try to conserve as much energy as possible for the body to use. Stress and worry can cause blood sugar to drop even though food may have been eaten at regular intervals, thus depleting the body's energy. In order to help your body heal itself, practise the art of relaxation and avoid stressful situations whenever possible.

One last point about blood sugar. Many individuals feel that their bodies need something sweet. They say that they have a sweet tooth or feel that a meal is not a meal without a pudding. As far as I'm concerned, there are two main reasons why we crave sweet things. One is because the blood sugar is low (this should not be the case once *Cooking Without* is put into practice); the second is because sweet foods are often used as a love substitute. This means that we work hard and push our bodies or give ourselves a hard time mentally by thinking about what we should be doing rather than treating ourselves with respect and kindness. Having punished ourselves, we suddenly crave something sweet in order to give back to ourselves. The fact that this sweet food often makes us feel worse, either because our blood sugar dips or because we feel guilty, causes a vicious circle to be set up. If you continue to crave sweet foods after putting this diet into practice, there may be an emotional problem, which needs to be addressed (see Emotions, addictions and ill health, page 18).

Migraines and Headaches

The pounding headaches which are one of the symptoms of migraines are caused by blood vessels in the brain becoming abnormally dilated.

This happens when serotonin levels in the body are low. Serotonin is a nerve transmitter which allows nerves to pass on messages to contract or dilate blood vessels. One of the main causes of low serotonin levels is low blood sugar. Interestingly, magnesium, which is the main mineral needed for serotonin production, is also the main mineral needed to detoxify the liver in order that the liver can support the blood sugar.

Essentially migraines and headaches are a low blood sugar problem (see page 3). It is therefore important for any headache or migraine sufferer to find out what is causing their blood sugar to drop so that they are able to prevent attacks.

Some individuals suffer migraine attacks when they don't eat sufficient food to keep their blood sugar stable. Going too long without eating can have a similar effect. Eating food to which one is intolerant causes a stress on the body, which in turn causes the blood sugar to drop. Chocolate, oranges, red wine and cheese have often been blamed for migraines but not everyone will have a problem with these foods. They may, however, have a problem with other foods. When sick, tired or under stress the body will react more strongly than when it is feeling well, so a food which causes a migraine one day may not do so if tested another day. Similarly if the blood sugar is well supported because a good meal has just been consumed the body may cope with the effects of an allergen. However, if the offending food is eaten on an empty stomach or when the blood sugar is low its impact will be greater.

Food is not the only stress that can cause the blood sugar to drop. Any stress on the body can cause the blood sugar and therefore the serotonin levels to drop and thus encourage a migraine or headache. Even though food may have been eaten to support the blood sugar, stress is capable of causing it to plummet quite rapidly. Emotional upheavals, anxiety, tension, bright lights, loud noises, travelling, dehydration, high toxin levels etc. can all be responsible. People react differently to different stresses.

Many people suffer from migraines at the weekend or at the start of a holiday, which seems very unfair. However, if you look at the circumstances you will see why. These days there is a tendency for individuals to live on their adrenalin (see blood sugar and Chronic Fatigue) especially when at work or when extra busy such as during the run up to a holiday. Adrenalin causes blood sugar to be released from the cells enabling us to live on our reserve supplies. When we stop being busy, for instance on a Saturday morning or when the holiday starts, our blood sugar drops because the adrenalin is not flowing. Until we have recovered some energy and our liver can support our blood sugar, we feel the effects of it being too low, and suffer from a headache or migraine.

A similar effect can sometimes be caused by people drinking lots of tea or coffee whilst at work. Both these substances kick the adrenal glands into producing blood sugar. Saturday morning arrives and you haven't had your usual coffee for the day and suddenly a headache starts to develop. Having a lie in at the weekend or when on holiday can add to the above problem or can cause a headache or migraine in its own right. If you are normally up and having breakfast by 7 to 8am and suddenly it's 11am and you haven't eaten, your blood sugar will be very low.

Many women have a migraine headache around the time of their period. What happens during a period is that the hormones, oestrogen and progesterone, drop before bleeding can start. This drop in hormone levels causes a drop in blood sugar levels. In many women this will cause them to feel more hungry, crave sweets, feel tired, irritable etc. – all low-blood-sugar symptoms; others will develop a headache or migraine.

The menopause is another time when the blood sugar becomes lower and many women who have never had a problem with headaches or migraines may suffer from them in their 40s. The menopause is causing a drop in hormones on a more permanent basis and until the body adjusts to these lower levels they can cause a problem.

Some drugs have been found to cause migraines. Occasionally it is the drugs used to counteract the headaches or migraines that are the problem. The pill is also a possible factor. All drugs hit the liver as the liver is the main organ of detoxification, but interestingly the liver is also the organ responsible for supporting the blood sugar. The liver and gall bladder meridian runs up each side of the neck vertebrae, over the top of the head and to the temples. Migraine headaches are often felt along one or both of these meridians.

The only other cause of headaches and migraines that I have met in practice and that seems unrelated to blood sugar levels is structural in origin. It could be anything from a bad bite, poor posture, or a body which is out of line through accidental damage. If you feel that this could be your problem then consult the relevant therapist, such as an osteopath or dentist.

Headaches and migraines are not a problem which we just have to learn to live with. There is always a reason and sometimes more than one reason for their presence. If we remove the cause then the body does not need to produce a headache or migraine to let us know that something is wrong. Eating as outlined in *Cooking Without* means that not only is food used to support the blood sugar but also many of the situations and substances which result in low blood sugar are avoided. Migraines and headaches can thus be alleviated whilst work is done on improving blood sugar levels on a more permanent basis.

Candida Albicans and Leaky Gut Syndrome

Inside our intestinal tract are minute organisms called intestinal flora. These bacteria are responsible, in part, for the absorption of nutrients and the elimination of waste products. Among the bacteria both good and bad exist, but normally the bad bacteria do not cause us any problems provided we have sufficient natural defences and good bacteria to keep them in their place. Nowadays, one particular bacteria called Candida Albicans is being encouraged to get out of hand and its overgrowth can cause a lot of problems.

This overgrowth is being caused by the way we eat, the over consumption of meat, sugar and refined carbohydrates, excess alcohol and a lack of fibre-rich foods, such as vegetables and complex carbohydrates. This over consumption, as well as feeding Candida, upsets the acid alkaline balance in the intestines, which in turn provides an ideal environment for its growth. Chlorine in our water supplies encourages Candida, as does the widespread use of the pill, antibiotics and hormones (either taken as medication or consumed in meat products). A further factor that is crucial in encouraging Candida overgrowth is a diminished function of the immune system which is certainly encouraged by our polluted, nutrient-deficient and stressful Western lifestyle.

Poor digestion encourages Candida as it allows food to travel too far down the digestive tract without being completely broken down. The food then provides nourishment for the Candida rather than for us. If insufficient hydrochloric acid is produced in the stomach the environment will not be sterile and therefore Candida and other bacteria can survive. A lack of hydrochloric acid also prevents the activation of the entire cascade of digestive enzymes. Poor digestion is often the reason why individuals may eat a food one day and feel fine, yet the next day they will develop Candida symptoms. There is a tendency to think that they must have an intolerance to the foodstuff when really it is the digestion which is varying. Digestion is hampered by *dampness*. In Chinese medicine individuals suffering from Candida would be considered to be too *damp.*

Dampness is encouraged by certain foods and there is a list of some, which promote dampness, in the section on allergies and intolerances and in *Vegetarian Cooking Without.* Digestion can be assisted by avoiding too many cold and damp foods, by chewing well, drinking an adequate supply of water to produce sufficient digestive juices (but not with meals) and taking a supplement of betaine hydrochloride or digestive enzymes if necessary. Certain bitter herbs are also well known digestive stimulants (ask in your local health food shop).

If Candida is allowed to overgrow it develops into a mycelial fungal form, which punctures the gut wall. This wall, which is normally very particular about what it allows through, is now open to absorb larger particles, such as food which has not been completely digested, toxins from the gut or from Candida metabolism and Candida itself. Any molecule crossing the gut wall into the blood stream will be 'inspected' by the immune system to assess whether the incoming material is safe or a foreign invader. Large undigested food molecules will elicit an immune response where antibodies are produced to counter an attack. This is the start of allergies and intolerances. The immune system which is over burdened with toxins and often suffering from a lack of nutrients is further weakened by having to defend itself. Candida is then more able to spread unhampered into the body.

Once Candida has broken through the gut wall we have a problem called leaky gut syndrome, where instead of the gut being the point of fuel or nutrient entry, it becomes a toxic factory allowing undesirable substances to penetrate into the body causing ill health. If the gut is unhealthy then so is the rest of the body. Leaky gut syndrome is thought to have a part to play in many major immune-related diseases such as Chronic Fatigue Syndrome, Rheumatoid arthritis, Lupus, Multiple Sclerosis, Psoriasis and Crohn's disease. It has also been implicated in autism and many other chronic ailments. Leaky gut syndrome puts added pressure on the liver, as its detoxification pathways are subsequently overloaded. There are other factors which are known to encourage a leaky gut besides Candida. They include alcohol, detergents, NSAIDs – or non steroidal anti inflammatory drugs (ie. aspirin and ibuprofen) – and organisms such as helicobacter.

Below is a list of symptoms which can be attributed to Candida overgrowth. You will notice that some of the symptoms also fit into the list of hypoglycaemia symptoms on page 4. Low blood sugar is a common forerunner of Candida problems.

Cystitis, thrush, urinary frequency, fungal infections, PMT, endometriosis, abdominal bloating, indigestion, heartburn, flatulence, diarrhoea, constipation, alternating diarrhoea and constipation, bad breath, dry or sore mouth, postnasal drip, acne, numbness, burning, tingling, itching, recurrent sore throats, pain or tightness in the chest, fluid in the ears, blurred vision, spots in front of the eyes, lethargy, mood swings, anxiety, irritability, depression, muscle aches, headaches, muzziness, dizziness, lack of concentration, memory lapses.

As can be seen from the above list, Candida Albicans merits attention, but all too frequently the attention is directed obsessively at killing the Candida without reference to the individual's body which has allowed the invasion to take place. Candida is present in all of us and can never be completely eliminated. Therefore working in isolation in trying to kill or starve the Candida means that as soon as treatment stops, it will thrive again. The emphasis should go on strengthening the body by detoxifying the cells and replenishing its mineral and vitamin reserves. This in turn will strengthen the immune system enabling it to overcome any invaders. Work also needs to be done on improving the digestion, repopulating the gut with friendly flora and healing the gut walls.

Too many Candida diets cause individuals to starve themselves by excessively limiting foods. For instance, many Candida regimes remove carbohydrates completely. This is based on the theory that carbohydrates convert to sugar and sugar feeds Candida. However, limiting carbohydrates encourages toxic symptoms as toxins are released from the cells in response to fasting (hardly eating) or a diet which is high in vegetables and low in carbohydrates

In order for this toxicity to be removed, the body needs energy (blood sugar) to work the elimination system. It also needs a medium which will soak up the acid waste or toxicity and remove it from the body. Complex carbohydrates are the only foods which fulfil these two roles. What is frequently termed 'die–off' in many Candida books and is supposedly caused by Candida dying and releasing its toxicity is, as far as I am concerned, a build up of toxins caused by eating insufficient quantities of the right kind of food. It happens to anyone who limits the quantity of food (especially carbohydrates) which they eat when detoxifying, whether they suffer from Candida or other problems. It can also be avoided.

The regime outlined in this book is ideal for Candida sufferers, even though it is high in carbohydrates. These carbohydrates are complex in form and will be tolerated by all except a very small minority who have intolerances to rice, millet etc. The rest of the diet is made up of vegetables, beans and pulses, and small amounts of meat or fish and eggs for those to whom these are acceptable. Fresh fruit needs to be severely limited and may need to be avoided in the early stages of treatment. Wheat and dairy produce are best avoided.

Foods which contain yeast, moulds or fungi such as dried fruit, mushrooms, shoyu/tamari/soya sauce, alcohol, yeast, yeast extract, bread, stock cubes, citric acid, monosodium glutamate, vinegar and cheese are generally recommended to be avoided by Candida patients. Whether or not this is the case will depend on whether or not the individual has an allergy or intolerance to yeast or an allergy or intolerance to any of these particular foods. If there is an allergy then even a small amount of the substance may cause a problem for the individual concerned. With intolerances it is more a question of the amount consumed. If the food is well digested I feel that many Candida sufferers can tolerate small amounts of the more acceptable of these foods, for instance dried fruit or mushrooms. A problem only develops if too much is eaten, or the food is not digested well and reaches the Candida. Only trial and error will really determine which foods you can include and the quantity. Often a food is better tolerated in the morning or lunch time when the digestion is less tired. Try avoiding all yeast-related products for at least three weeks or until symptoms subside, then test a small amount of yeast-based food two times in one day. If symptoms return then there is a problem and the food needs removing for a longer period of time. Eventually, when health has returned, foods which originally caused problems should be able to be re-introduced.

On an emotional level, Candida sufferers are lacking in self worth and are very hard on themselves (see 'Emotions, Addictions and Ill Health', page 18). Even if they are not trying to be Superman or Super-woman they still push and expect too much of their bodies. The reasons that cause Candida sufferers to be so hard on themselves will be uncovered as detoxification takes place. These reasons, which can be termed 'emotional toxicity', will be released and eliminated along with the physical toxins present in the body.

Allergies and Intolerances

Very few people suffer from allergies, many more suffer from intolerances. Allergies cause obvious symptoms such as swellings and rashes. Intolerances have a much more subtle effect, undermining health but not necessarily causing immediate or obvious symptoms. Foods or substances to which intolerances develop tend to be the ones we come into contact with on a regular basis, such as wheat and milk. Individuals can get hooked on the food causing them problems and so will crave and temporarily feel better for eating this substance. However, once it is removed from their diet, they will notice tremendous improvements in their health and well being.

At the heart of all allergies and intolerances, whether caused by food or other irritants, is our body's own defence system. The immune system is a complex army of cells, which protect the body from external invaders. When working harmoniously the immune system protects us from many micro-organisms, some of which cause infectious diseases.

Candida and Leaky Gut Syndrome are often responsible for the immune system being invaded (see page 8). They cause the intestinal wall to develop large leaky spaces, which in turn allow partly digested food and toxins to reach the immune system. The immune system produces antibodies to tag these foreign invaders and will then deposit them in the body in areas of least resistance such as in the skin, soft tissue or joints. Protective cells underneath the skin and under every lining in the body are triggered by the antibodies in the blood to defend the body. They believe themselves to be under attack and switch to a protective mode by launching a chemical attack on the invader and oozing out histamine and other substances. This creates inflammation around the invader in order that it can be engulfed. The liver is the organ which produces anti-histamine to counteract the swelling and inflammation. If however the liver is congested with fats and toxins it may not be providing a good anti-histamine service and hence the inflammation remains. This can cause irritation and soreness but it can also be the cause of fluid and weight gain and be responsible for many health problems. A lack of water or dehydration encourages the release of excess histamine and is therefore another factor which may be implicated in food reactions.

The antibodies produced by the immune system in order to tag the invaders and signal the body to produce histamine, are known as the Ig antibodies. There are two types of Ig antibodies, IgG and IgE. With the classic IgE reaction there is an exaggerated histamine response, causing a quick onset of symptoms from within a minute to two hours. A single factor such as dust, fur or seafood is usually responsible. Even a minor exposure can trigger an immense, maybe life-threatening reaction. This is a true allergy and once triggered an IgE allergy is often permanent though tremendous improvements can occur after detoxification.

IgG reactions are quite different and can be regarded as intolerances rather than allergies. Symptoms can occur in almost any organ or tissue of the body and they can take from several hours to several days to appear thus making the link with what we have eaten, or been in contact with, more difficult to determine. With IgG reactions it is a question of quantity, you may be intolerant to cows' milk but if you only have a little you may not respond. Also the B lymphocytes which set up IgG reactions only have a memory time of 2 to 3 months. If you withdraw a food for 3 months they forget it and you can often go back to eating it provided you have healed the condition which caused the problem in the first place.

Although the issue is food intolerance, it is not really the food but other factors which are the main problem. Every food is a potential allergen if not properly broken down by the digestive system. The ability of the stomach to make hydrochloric acid is important as a lack of this prevents food from being properly digested. In Chinese medicine allergies are related to a state of *dampness* in the body. The digestion can be likened to a fire burning and too much damp energy in the body or in the food being digested will prevent the fire from completely burning the fuel.

If food that has not been properly digested passes too far into the intestines the result is putrefaction instead of digestion. The environment is then perfect for the growth of yeast and fungi such as Candida, who have food to eat and a warm damp environment to live in. Although we all have Candida present it will not be encouraged to grow and take over if the environment is not to its liking. The main foods which encourage dampness include, wheat, sugar, honey, dairy produce (milk, cheese, ice cream, yogurt), eggs, fatty meat especially beef and pork, butter, oil, fried food, nut butters, fruit juice especially citrus, bananas and tomatoes. If you look at the above list it contains many of the foods which most people live on – especially children.

Food intolerances or allergies cause a drop in blood sugar levels, (see blood sugar, page 3) which in turn, causes a lack of energy. This lack of energy not only affects us in our daily lives but affects all our internal organs and systems such as digestion, immune system, detoxification etc. We thus have a vicious circle, low blood sugar creating a lack of energy, weakening the digestion and immune system encouraging more intolerances and producing low blood sugar. The problem foods therefore need removing and the blood sugar needs raising by eating regular meals. Sometimes, when the blood sugar drops in response to an allergy or intolerance the adrenal glands kick in to produce adrenalin which causes an emergency supply of blood sugar to be released from the cells. This can cause, for instance, the hyperactive behaviour seen in children who are intolerant of certain foods, drinks or additives.

With food allergies and intolerances it is obviously sensible to remove the offending foods and there are many therapists specialising in allergy testing (see index). However, if the offending foods are removed, but there is no emphasis on improving health, then often further foods will start to cause problems. Detoxification is important, as is replenishing the vitamin and mineral reserves in the body. Only by getting the wrong things out and the right things in can the body and its systems function optimally. Detoxification also helps to remove emotional toxicity, which can have a large part to play in allergies and intolerances. In *Vegetarian Cooking Without* I cover the emotional reasons for such problems in more depth. Work also needs to be done on improving digestion, raising the blood sugar, replacing good intestinal flora and healing the intestinal walls. *Cooking Without* will assist the building of good health.

Once health has been improved foods which initially caused problems can be reintroduced. If you introduce them too soon you may find that you react to them more strongly than you did before. This is because, having removed them, the body has lost its ability to adapt or cope. Do not worry about this and continue working on improving your health; all but foods responsible for severe allergies will eventually be accepted. Never introduce more than one new food at a time and do not overeat new foods, even if you can tolerate them.

Irritable Bowel Syndrome

Irritable bowel syndrome (IBS) is not a disease so much as a label used to cover a collection of symptoms. It is given when the results of medical investigations are negative – in other words there is no serious disease present, but there is no explanation for what is causing the symptoms.

Symptoms of IBS can include flatulence, abdominal pain, abdominal bloating, diarrhoea, constipation or alternating bouts of both. Diarrhoea can be urgent, especially first thing in the mornings, and there may be mucous in the stools. If IBS is not a disease then we need to look at the symptoms present to see what the body is trying to tell us.

Irritable bowel syndrome can be a symptom of poor digestion even though the individuals concerned may feel that they digest well and do not have a problem with indigestion or heartburn. Poor digestion can be caused by food intolerances, having low levels of stomach acid or digestive enzymes, being too cold and damp, or as a result of stress. In turn, poor digestion leads to an overgrowth of bad intestinal flora.

Food intolerances are very common with IBS sufferers. Wheat, yeast and dairy produce are some of the main offenders, but any foodstuff can be responsible. Bran, which is often recommended for sufferers, often makes IBS worse. This is especially so if the individual has an intolerance to wheat, but bran is also capable of causing irritation to the bowel lining.

Low levels of stomach acid or digestive enzymes prevent food being completely broken down and digested. This means that partly digested food travels too far down the digestive tract where it provides food for the growth of unfriendly bacteria such as Candida. Candida is usually part of the problem with IBS sufferers and can be responsible for flatulence and bloating as well as irregular bowel motions. In order to discourage Candida the diet may need adjusting (see Candida, page 8), the gut needs repopulating with friendly flora and the digestion needs to be improved so that the main substance reaching the lower intestines is the fibre left over from food.

Digestion is affected by stress. When the adrenalin flows, as it does when an individual is under stress, the body prepares for a 'flight or fight' situation. During this period the body slows down any non-essential processes and concentrates on sending energy to the limbs and brain. As digestion is not really necessary when fighting or fleeing, this is one of the processes which slows down. Because stress is such an integral part of most people's lives nowadays, individuals are often unaware that they are stressed – it's the way they have always been.

Digestion is also affected by a general lack of energy. As most people these days have low blood sugar problems and, therefore, a lack of energy it is difficult for any body functions to operate optimally. If we are tired so are our processes of digestion and elimination.

Cold and dampness affect digestion. Viewed from a Chinese perspective if the digestion is too cold and damp it will not burn the fuel or food and will therefore provide nourishment for Candida. Diarrhoea, especially first thing in the morning, alternating constipation and diarrhoea and mucous in the stools, are all symptoms of cold and damp. In *Vegetarian Cooking Without,* I explain Chinese medicine in a little more depth and also list foods which are warming and foods which remove damp. There are also numerous books on Chinese medicine if you wish to further your knowledge in this area of investigation. A good idea is to consume a drink of warming herbs and spices such as ginger, cinnamon, fennel and liquorice, approximately half an hour before eating to warm and assist the digestion. It is also sensible to avoid too many raw, cold foods.

Drugs, especially antibiotics, often have a part to play in IBS symptoms. Antibiotics kill off good intestinal flora and encourage the bad to proliferate. It takes time to repopulate the gut after a course of antibiotics and for the body to regain its integrity. Overuse of antibiotics will need a longer period of cleansing and healing.

Irritable bowel syndrome, as you can see, is not something that has to be accepted and lived with. There are reasons for its presence and, therefore, there are solutions. Following a *Cooking Without* regime should help considerably.

Chronic Fatigue (ME) and TATT (Tired All The Time)

Chronic fatigue is not always what it seems to be. Those who accept that it exists are usually looking to blame a virus. However, the virus is irrelevant as many people with Chronic fatigue symptoms do not have a virus present, and many with the virus present are fit and healthy. Many individuals with Chronic fatigue are sick because their immune systems have been weakened, making them prey to any virus which comes along. It is of no use trying to find the magic bullet which will kill the virus but more a matter of looking at why the immune system has been compromised and then working at strengthening it.

Candida weakens the body and the immune system, and many Chronic fatigue sufferers have Candida present. The body and immune system can also be weakened by stress, by poor nutrition and by general toxicity, whether it be from a toxic-laden diet, drug abuse or environmental pollution. Antibiotic overuse and vaccinations are also frequent forerunners of Chronic fatigue.

Chronic fatigue has been referred to as 'yuppie flu', and it is no coincidence that ambitious over-achievers are susceptible to the problem. Like most Chronic fatigue sufferers, they have been living on adrenalin and pushing their bodies for too long. They may get up feeling tired, but once into the swing of the day, the adrenalin starts to flow and they feel fine. Later, when the energy flags, a game of squash or a three-mile jog gives their adrenal glands another kick and they are ready for a busy evening. Add to this the type of lifestyle that many young people live – eating too much junk food, missing meals, partaking of alcohol, taking the pill, taking antibiotics for infections – and you can see how eventually the body inevitably gives in. The mother who works, or the over-stressed businessman, may not have the glamorous lifestyle of the yuppie, but the effects of living on adrenalin are the same. Chronic fatigue is not a disease but a series of symptoms which the body is using as a signal to let the individual know that all is not well. In fact, everything is exhausted.

Chronic fatigue can be seen at one end of the scale in individuals who generally do not feel well, but cope each day with a multitude of minor health problems and a continual lack of energy. They struggle by living on adrenalin and pushing their bodies to keep going. These individuals are on the verge of Chronic fatigue, and it only takes a strong antibiotic from the doctor, a dose of flu or a severely stressful situation to push them over the edge. At the other end of the scale are those Chronic fatigue sufferers who are so sick and weak they can barely stand up. They may ache from head to toe, find it impossible to think or concentrate, feel permanently sick or dizzy, and will have many more individual symptoms.

In order to recover from Chronic fatigue, work needs to be done on raising the blood sugar levels. This relieves some of the symptoms which are due to low blood sugar (see page 3) and takes pressure off the exhausted adrenal glands. The dietary regime outlined in this book is ideal for this. Chronic fatigue is similar to Candida in that it cannot be treated as an isolated problem without the individual being taken into consideration. Work needs to be done on detoxifying the body and replacing lost minerals in an attempt to repair and support all the organs, glands and systems which have become implicated. The issue of self-worth needs consideration because a lack of it is frequently the motivator for over-achievement (see Emotions, Addictions and Ill Health, below)

Emotions, Addictions and Ill Health

Addictions are very common in our society and range from the more acceptable ones, such as sugar or chocolate addictions, to the more severe drug and alcohol-based ones. In between is a selection, which includes, among many others, addictive spending, smoking, gambling, sex and shoplifting.

What each of these addictions does is to make us feel better temporarily. The fact that the consequences might be injurious to us is irrelevant at the time; we know that we will feel better if we have a chocolate bar, find a new lover, buy ourselves a new stereo or have a drink, but what we are actually doing is avoiding facing the reality of our situation. When we come down from the high that addictions create, we often feel worse than before. Unless individuals find the reasons why they are addicted they will not recover, or they will swap one addiction for another.

Within each of us is a male and female side of our personality – the *animus* and *anima* (see chart, below). The animus, or male psyche, used positively is responsible for drive, ambition, determination, self-reliance and discipline. The female anima used positively is responsible for feelings, emotions, intuition, softness and caring.

Some females have a strong animus or male side and would not be happy staying at home. They want to be out there in the world of work. Similarly, some men who have a strong anima to contend with are not assertive enough to work in the world of business but are happy in the

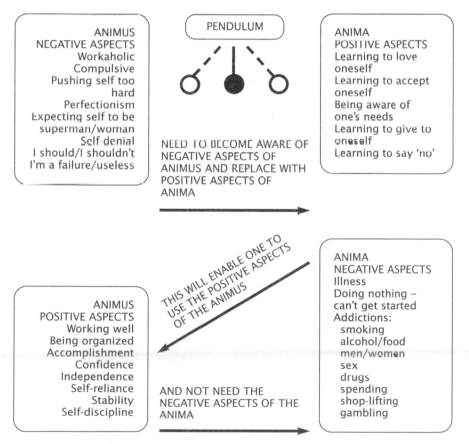

ANIMUS
NEGATIVE ASPECTS
Workaholic
Compulsive
Pushing self too hard
Perfectionism
Expecting self to be superman/woman
Self denial
I should/I shouldn't
I'm a failure/useless

PENDULUM

ANIMA
POSITIVE ASPECTS
Learning to love oneself
Learning to accept oneself
Being aware of one's needs
Learning to give to oneself
Learning to say 'no'

NEED TO BECOME AWARE OF NEGATIVE ASPECTS OF ANIMUS AND REPLACE WITH POSITIVE ASPECTS OF ANIMA

THIS WILL ENABLE ONE TO USE THE POSITIVE ASPECTS OF THE ANIMUS

ANIMUS
POSITIVE ASPECTS
Working well
Being organized
Accomplishment
Confidence
Independence
Self-reliance
Stability
Self-discipline

ANIMA
NEGATIVE ASPECTS
Illness
Doing nothing –
can't get started
Addictions:
    smoking
    alcohol/food
    men/women
    sex
    drugs
    spending
    shop-lifting
    gambling

AND NOT NEED THE NEGATIVE ASPECTS OF THE ANIMA

The Animus and Anima Chart

caring professions or at home with the children. What is important is that we learn to be true to ourselves and find our own balance between the anima and animus. If, however, we have been brought up to suppress one side of our personality or overemphasize the other, then often illness or addictive behaviour takes over to try and create a balance.

This affects mostly those individuals who have an innately strong feminine side which they have learnt to repress or hide. Those with an innately strong masculine side will fit more easily into the roles which parents and society deem acceptable.

Upbringing has a lot to do with the way we are. Parents have often taught their offspring not to be selfish or acknowledge their own needs (religion may have encouraged this). This lack of self-acknowledgement may have been passed on by parents who had problems. Perhaps they could not express their emotions, and in doing so inadvertently taught the child to hide its feelings, or perhaps the child received very little attention so that it only felt acknowledged when it did something exceptional. Thus it always had to drive itself hard and aim continually higher in order to gain a reward. Whatever the background and this can be as varied as the individuals with the problems, what is unfortunately being taught is a lack of self worth. The feminine side, which enables us to love, cherish and be kind to ourselves, is suppressed, and the masculine side is encouraged, becomes overdeveloped and expresses itself negatively. Thus, instead of working well, individuals become workaholics; instead of being self-disciplined, they become self-denying; instead of being organized, they become perfectionists. Each person finds their own way of validating their self-worth depending on their individual talents. Others will turn this drive inwards and will just be hard on themselves by saying – 'I'm a failure' or 'I'm useless'.

In the middle of the chart is a pendulum which will always find a person's true balance between their masculine and feminine sides. If the pendulum has swung too far to the left because an individual has been working too hard or expecting too much of themselves, then it will need to swing excessively to the right to rebalance. If they are able to compensate by being kind and giving to themselves, then all will be well, but what happens if they have run out of time or have never been taught to love and nurture themselves?

Addictions and illness become an alternative that satisfies a deep yearning within the subconscious. After a hard day individuals may turn to food, alcohol or sex in order to try to rebalance. Similarly, being ill means that they are forced to give themselves time and attention or allow others to do this by nursing them better. The feminine side may be lived out through illness or addictions, but unless we own it ourselves, then peace, health and happiness will never be fully attained.

In order to rebalance the feminine and masculine it is first necessary for individuals to see how these two aspects of their psyche are being used in their lives. Being aware of when and how they are using the negative animus is the first step. All individuals who are ill or have addictions have far higher expectations of themselves than they do of anyone else. A good way to think of it is as a shadow self, walking behind you with a whip, always pushing and tormenting and expecting more. Once one realizes how and when the whip is being used, it is much easier not to expect yourself to be superman or superwoman.

Rebuilding the positive side of the anima is about learning to be kind to oneself, to give and to indulge oneself. It is the process of learning to understand one's needs, to love, nurture and accept oneself despite any imperfections, and this is the basis of developing real self-worth.

A good idea is to write a list of 20 positive ways to give to oneself. Individuals who indulge themselves with sweets, alcohol or spending, for example, often feel really bad and are hard on themselves for doing so (the animus again). These new ways are all about invoking feelings of 'this is nice', 'this is for me', 'I deserve this'. The list will vary from person to person, for what makes one of us feel indulgent will not do the same for another. It is not the issue that is important, it is the feelings of love we invoke when we do these things that we are trying to foster. The list can include things as simple as: a pot of tea with time to sit and savour it; a lazy bath; an early night; reading; walking; looking at the view; watching the cat; buying oneself a bunch of flowers.

Some individuals may say, 'Oh that's not me. I always buy myself presents, have an early night etc.', but often they are doing these things for the wrong reasons. Are they buying new clothes because they deserve them or because their self-worth is invested in looking good?

Are they indulging in an early night because they feel they would like it or to escape from reality?

By learning to be kind to ourselves we gradually discover that we have needs and that these needs must be met if we are to stay healthy. We also need to love ourselves sufficiently to prioritize these needs in our life and to have enough self-worth to be able to say 'no' when others try to distract us. An example of this might be someone who needs their own space but who has a partner and family who are clingy and always demanding attention. Rather than feeling like a bad person who must be a failure and must work harder at their marriage and relationships, this person needs to accept that this is the way they are, that freedom is one of their needs and must be satisfied.

Although this all seems very indulgent and selfish, so is being ill or addicted. It is far better to give oneself the time, attention and love while one is still able, rather than keep denying oneself and eventually needing to be looked after.

Because the male animus is overdeveloped, it is easy to turn indulgences into animus things. For instance, we may say to ourselves, 'I'm going to read my book tonight', but instead of doing it with love we do it with the whip, 'You will find time to read that book'. Suddenly it has changed from a feminine, caring action into a driving ambition. In this instance, it is better to swap what we intended doing for something else: 'Instead of the book, which I'm too tired to read, I'm going to have an early night'.

Eventually, we can stop the pendulum swinging so wildly and decrease our need for addictions and illness by learning to live out the positive sides of the anima and animus. Following the diet outlined in *Cooking Without* will assist in this process. Because this eating regime is designed to detoxify, it will help you to work through mental and emotional toxicity which may have caused you to use the negative expressions of the anima and animus. Individuals who have worked on themselves in this way are then able to tap into the feminine qualities of feeling and intuition to see their path in life more clearly. The new base of confidence and self-reliance which they have created by utilizing the very positive attributes of the animus, will then enable them to move forward along this path more easily.

Anorexia and Bulimia

Anorexia and bulimia are the result of mental and emotional toxicity, which in turn affects the physical body. If you look at the animus and anima chart (page 19) you will be able to see where they fit in. Anorexia fits in the top, left hand corner with the negative aspects of the animus. Bulimia fits in the bottom, right hand corner with the negative aspects of the anima. Individuals who suffer from both anorexia and bulimia have a pendulum swinging wildly between the two extremes.

Anorexics are very hard on themselves; they deny themselves food and they feel that they are too fat. They are usually perfectionists who have high expectations of themselves and they push themselves severely to reach their goals. They live in their heads and are controlled by what they think they should and shouldn't do. They have lost touch with how they feel and are very unforgiving of themselves. Bulimia takes over when the pendulum swings. When the body cannot stand anymore harshness, and is crying out deep inside for love and attention, the bulimic will binge. Others who don't turn to food may turn to sex, shopping or other addictions. However, whatever they turn to will never fill the bottomless pit which is deep inside of them, for it can never be filled with external fixes. They don't love themselves and no-one else and nothing else can ever fill the gap. Bulimics will eventually feel the guilt and horror of what they have done and will swing back to the negative animus. They will start being hard on themselves again and will make themselves sick. Those who have used other love substitutes will be similarly hard on themselves over the money they have spent or the individual they have slept with.

Anorexics and bulimics need to learn to love themselves before they can learn to have a healthy relationship with food. If they are force fed until they gain weight, as so often happens, this will only deepen their problems. The outside appearance is only a mirror of what is going on inside and it is the internal issues which need dealing with in order for the anorexic to cope with gaining weight.

I find that the *Cooking Without* regime works well with anorexics and bulimics as, once they realise that they can eat as much as they like but that they don't put on weight easily, they are happy to stay with the regime. Not only does the diet build health it also detoxifies any mental and emotional toxicity which is at the root of their problems. If they can then be helped through this period with counselling, by the time they start to gain weight they will be ready to cope with this.

Why Gluten-Free, Yeast-Free, Sugar-Free, Saturated Fat-Free and Dairy-Free?

Gluten and Wheat

Wheat as a dietary constituent has some advantages, but on the whole these are outweighed by its disadvantages. Wheat is generally thought of as a wholesome, nutritious, fibre-rich food. Unfortunately, for many individuals (including many who do not realize), wheat is actually causing them problems.

Wheat contains gluten which, when wet, is a sticky glue-like substance. Not long ago, flour and water were used as cheap glue. In our gut this glue can play havoc with the digestion and absorption of nutrients. Because gluten is so sticky and difficult to digest, it encourages the growth of unfriendly bacteria (see Candida, page 8) which are responsible for producing toxic substances and gas. Constipation, diarrhoea, bloatedness, indigestion, flatulence and wind are all problems which can benefit from the removal of wheat from the diet.

Wheat is one of the most common foods to which people become intolerant. It can make an individual feel tired, irritable and depressed, as well as aggravating other diseases, such as arthritis, psoriasis and eczema. Because most people eat wheat so often, the body adapts and copes, and they are unaware that it does not agree with them (see Allergies and Intolerances, page 12). Once it is removed from the diet, however, many individuals notice tremendous improvements in their health and well being.

Wheat has a suppressive action on the liver, so even individuals who seem to tolerate wheat well actually slow down their rate of elimination by eating wheat too often. Wheat is therefore best avoided in the early stages of elimination, especially if your health is seriously below par. After working on the eating regime outlined in this book to a point where you feel fit and healthy, try including wheat again, but never include it in large quantities and never more than once per day. Spelt is a form of wheat, which is derived from an ancient grain, and although it is not gluten free, it seems to cause fewer problems than modern wheat.

Other grains that contain gluten are rye, oats and barley, and although some individuals may tolerate these better than wheat, others may need to avoid them completely until their health has improved.

Dairy Produce

MILK

Milk has an image of being the perfect food but it is perfect only when fed from the mother to her infant. A young child eventually loses the enzyme necessary to digest milk, and after this stage, milk becomes acid and mucous-forming, capable of upsetting normal bowel flora and preventing the absorption of vitamins and minerals. Many individuals develop intolerances to milk and its products, and they are often unaware of this until milk is removed from the diet.

In general, we are led to believe that we do not obtain sufficient calcium and that milk and milk products are essential. However, calcium is readily available in foods such as vegetables, fruit, nuts and pulses. If there is a problem with inadequate calcium, it is far more likely to be through poor absorption than through poor intake, and it is more often the individuals who are intolerant of dairy produce who have the lowest calcium levels.

If you are unsure about your calcium levels it is best to consult a qualified nutritional therapist for advice on supplementation, particularly if you have an intolerance to dairy produce.

If diet and absorption are improved we can often live more healthily without milk. This can be seen in many tribal communities where milk and milk products are not consumed yet children grow well, producing good bones and teeth, and diseases such as arthritis and osteoporosis are unknown.

CHEESE

Cheese not only has the negative aspects of milk but it is also high in fat and salt and difficult to digest. Cottage cheese is more acceptable once health has been attained.

BUTTER

Butter is the fatty part of the milk. But because little of the milk remains, it can often be tolerated, even by individuals who are unable to tolerate milk. If a form of fat is used for spreading, I think that butter is preferable to the chemically derived margarines, but it should be used in moderation.

YOGURT

Live yogurt is the most favourable of all milk products due to the fact that it is low in fat and is partly digested by the action of the micro-organisms it contains. These micro-organisms assist in the re-population of the intestinal tract with friendly bacteria. Yogurt does, however, still carry the negative aspects of milk and is often better tolerated if made from sheep or goats' milk.

Fats and Oils

Fats and oils can be categorized into saturates, monounsaturates and polyunsaturates.

SATURATED FATS

These are the ones we are constantly being told to cut down on, and all the recipes in this book are free from added saturated fat. I feel, however, that the reason our bodies do not cope well nowadays with saturated fat is because we are so full of toxins and lacking in vitamins and minerals. The liver, which is our main organ of detoxification, is also the principal organ that deals with fat. If the liver is struggling to detoxify, it will also be struggling to cope with fat.

The liver is also the organ that balances the production of cholesterol in the body. Cholesterol is a fat which has gained a bad reputation as far as health is concerned, its excess being associated with conditions such as heart attacks and strokes. Cholesterol is necessary for many different body functions, however, and if we do not absorb sufficient amounts from our food, the liver is capable of making more. Equally, if we have too much cholesterol, the liver is capable of removing any excess by excreting it in the form of bile acids. In order to perform this cholesterol balancing act, the liver is dependent on obtaining an adequate supply of nutrients and energy from the diet. *Cooking Without* aims to supply these.

It is also important that we encourage a good bile flow. In order to do this we do need to eat some fat in the diet as bile is released in response to fat or oil being digested. Therefore, do not completely remove fat or oil from your diet.

As well as excess cholesterol, toxicity is released from the liver via the bile, and in order for both of these to be excreted from the body once they are in the digestive tract, adequate amounts of fibre are needed to assist their elimination. This prevents them from being reabsorbed into the body.

The diet outlined in this book enables an adequate intake of fat and plenty of fibre to be consumed. As far as I am concerned, the reason why our ancestors could eat a high-fat diet and not suffer from the rate of heart disease that afflicts modern society is that they had the necessary vitamins, minerals and fibre in their diets, and they were not overloaded with toxins.

It is best to limit saturated fats while detoxifying, but do not be obsessive about removing every scrap. People are often told not to eat eggs because they are high in fat and cholesterol, but eggs also contain lecithin, a fat emulsifier, and are quite acceptable used in sensible quantities. Even lean meat contains saturated fat, and so it is sensible to eat a varied diet which contains some fish and to have a number of vegetarian days. Although coconut is of vegetable origin, its oil is the highest in saturated fat of all vegetable oils, and so it should be used sparingly. Butter, I feel, is the most acceptable substance for spreading and is quite admissible if used in small quantities.

MONOUNSATURATED FATS

These include olive oil, and although little has been spoken of monounsaturates in the past, they are now being regarded as helpful fats in the diet (the Mediterranean diet contains plenty of olive oil). Olive oil is also the most stable oil when heated. All oil, however, becomes increasingly toxic when heated, so limit very hot frying. Do include some monounsaturated oil in your diet. Add olives to suitable recipes or eat them as a snack, or use olive oil in salad dressings or pour it over rice or vegetables.

POLYUNSATURATED FATS

We have been constantly encouraged to use these fats, but this is not necessarily a good idea. All oils contain essential fatty acids but linolenic acid is the essential fatty acid of which we are most in need. This is best obtained from eating fish (preferably oily), green leafy vegetables or from linseed oil and linseeds.

Unfortunately, if we eat too many polyunsaturates, linolenic acid is outweighed by the linoleic acid found in polyunsaturated oils, and this causes an imbalance in our bodies. Therefore, polyunsaturated oils are best used in moderation with fish, green vegetables and linseed oil being consumed to provide a balance. Most margarines are made from polyunsaturates, but they are also produced using chemicals and are then partly hydrogenated, which turns some of the polyunsaturates into saturated fat. The hydrogenation process also causes the production of free radicals (harmful substances) and changes the structure of the oil from a cis form to a trans form. This trans form is rarely found in nature and is therefore unacceptable to the human body. Avoid the use of margarine unless you cannot tolerate butter, in which case find one of the margarines which is not hydrogenated and is labelled high in cis form fatty acids.

Certain measures can be taken to safeguard the use of fats and oils in the diet:

1 Consume most oils in the form of foods, e.g. nuts, seeds, olives, beans, sweetcorn and linseeds.
2 Include some linseed oil in your daily diet to balance linoleic acid with linolenic acid. Linseeds can be bought from health-food shops and are pleasant to take, sprinkled on breakfast cereals, salads or in soups. Try taking 1–2 dessertspoons per day for a real health benefit. Linseed oil can be taken from the spoon or used in salad dressings.
3 Use cold-pressed oil, as heavily processed oil will have suffered oxidative and chemical damage.
4 Buy oil in small glass bottles and store in the fridge.
5 Improving nutrition will enable fats in any form to be more readily assimilated by the body.

Salt

Sodium is an essential mineral in the body, and together with potassium, magnesium and calcium, it forms one of the four bulk minerals. An over-consumption of salt upsets the delicate balance between these minerals, and the accumulation of sodium in the cells causes the latter to become more acidic. Other micro-minerals such as zinc and selenium, which the body may be deficient in, will not be readily absorbed unless the four bulk minerals are well balanced.

Our bodies do need some salt, as sodium is lost through the skin and faeces. Approximately half a gram per day is needed, and this small amount can be obtained by eating natural foods such as vegetables.

Salt is not the only form of sodium to enter our bodies. Other forms include monosodium glutamate (MSG, used as a flavour enhancer), sodium bicarbonate (used in baking powder), sodium nitrate and nitrite (used as preservatives), and hydrolysed proteins (used in stock cubes).

Avoid adding salt to your food for at least three to four months. You will then start to taste the food rather than the salt, and you will find that many of the previous things you ate are too salty. If salt is then needed in the occasional soup or casserole you will be able to add it in order to improve the taste. You should not need to put salt in cooked vegetables or grains or on the table.

Sugar

If we ate sugar in its natural form of fruit or sugar cane, there would be a limit to how much sugar we could consume. Along with sugar, we would obtain lots of fibre and the vitamins and minerals needed to digest the sugar. The fibre content means that it would take time to break down the structure and release the sugar into the bloodstream.

If, however, we eat manufactured sugar or products made from this (such as biscuits, cakes and sweets), we encourage low blood sugar or hypoglycaemia. This sudden surge of sugar into the bloodstream and its removal by the pancreas results in the roller coaster effects of cravings, highs and then lows, which leave us feeling physically, mentally and emotionally below par (see Low Blood Sugar, page 3). Sugar encourages the overgrowth of bad intestinal flora and should be avoided in all its forms. Brown sugar, although retaining some nutrients, still contains 97 per cent white sugar. When health has been attained, a little honey, molasses or no-sugar fruit spread is acceptable.

Yeast and Fermented Products

Because yeast-related products can aggravate Candida symptoms and upset the digestive tract, it is best to avoid these products on a temporary basis and then watch how your body reacts as you introduce them at a later date. These include yeast, yeast extract, vinegar, citric acid, monosodium glutamate, stock cubes, miso, shoyu/tamari/soya sauce, alcohol, cheese, mushrooms and dried fruit.

Some of these foods, such as mushrooms and dried fruit, will be acceptable to many Candida sufferers, if used sparingly. Some individuals will, however, have an intolerance to yeast and will need to remove all yeast and fermented products for a much longer period. See Candida Albicans (page 8) and Allergies and Intolerances (page 12).

Dos and Don'ts of Detoxification

It is difficult to devise a dietary regime that suits everyone, hence the flexible margins in this book regarding certain foods. It is probably best to err on the side of caution and remove any suspect food for a period of time or until an improvement in health has been achieved. Removing a substance from the diet means that our bodies lose their adaptability to that food, so that if it is causing a problem, this will become more apparent when it is reintroduced. When the toxins have eventually been removed from the body, the immune system will be stronger, and foods that originally caused problems can be included in the diet once again.

Meat

Meat should be eaten no more than twice a week. Choose organic produce where possible. Eat poultry and game in preference to lamb, but eat lamb in preference to beef and avoid pork. Processed and cured meat such as sausages, bacon and ham should be eliminated from the diet.

Fish

Eat fish up to three times a week, preferably a selection of oily as well as white fish. Do not eat smoked fish or reconstituted fish products, such as fish fingers. Frozen fish is acceptable if a fresh supply is unavailable. Tins of salmon, tuna, sardines and other fish can be used.

Eggs

Up to five eggs per week may be used, preferably organically produced. If you don't eat meat or fish you may use up to seven eggs per week. Those with allergies to eggs could try using an egg replacer in baked dishes (see 'Cooking Ingredients and Methods', page 37).

Dairy Produce

Avoid all milk – skimmed or whole, cream and cheese. Yogurt may be acceptable if health problems are not too severe, preferably made from sheep or goats' milk. Limit yourself to two to three servings per week.

Alternative Milks

Soya milk may be used in moderation, preferably made from organic soya beans, but without additives such as fruit sugars. Soya yogurt can be bought or made. Do not overuse soya milk as it is quite high in fat and difficult to digest. Rice, almond or other nut milks can be substituted if soya is not tolerated (see recipes).

Vegetables

Approximately 40 per cent of food consumed should be in the form of vegetables. Each day, aim to consume a large, varied salad and a good selection of cooked vegetables, as well as having at least two completely vegetarian days each week. Try to vary the vegetables as much as possible and use them when in season. If possible, buy organically grown produce.

Use vegetables such as: carrots, parsnips, turnips, swede, beetroot, celeriac, cabbage, Brussels sprouts, broccoli, cauliflower, kale, onions, leeks, celery, French beans, runner beans, peas, sweetcorn, marrow, pumpkin, courgettes, lettuce, Chinese leaves, radish, cress, fennel, watercress, endive, cucumber, sprouted seeds.

Peppers, aubergines, potatoes and tomatoes should be eaten sparingly because they contain more natural toxins than other vegetables. Limit mushrooms because they encourage the overgrowth of the yeast Candida albicans. Limit spinach, because it is high in oxalic acid which is capable of binding minerals such as calcium and preventing their absorption.

Beans and Pulses

These are good sources of protein, especially for vegetarians, and can be included in soups, casseroles and salads.

Nuts

Avoid salted nuts and peanuts. Use nuts in moderation, as they are high in oil and not easy to digest. Nuts are a good source of vegetable protein. Use mainly almonds, cashews, hazelnuts and walnuts. Use as snacks, in muesli, nut roasts and nut butters.

Seeds

Like nuts, seeds are a good source of vegetable protein. Use sesame, sunflower and pumpkin seeds and spreads such as tahini.

Rice

Rice is the ideal food for keeping blood sugar stable whilst soaking up toxic waste from the body. Preferably use short-grain, organically grown brown rice. You can use rice without limit, but each day aim to consume between 4–10 oz (115–285g (½–1½ cups) of rice, uncooked weight.

Buckwheat, Millet and Quinoa

These grains can be used instead of, or as well as, rice in the form of whole grains or flakes.

Corn

Corn can be used as a thickening agent and for baking in the form of flour and is available in an unbleached form in most health food shops. Corn can also be used as sweetcorn or popcorn. Some people do have allergies to corn. If this is the case, use substitutions for corn in the recipes.

Wheat

Wheat contains gluten so avoid all wheat products, such as bread, cakes, biscuits, pasta, cereals, and flour, for at least three months or for the duration of detoxification if health is still below par. When wheat is reintroduced, eat it no more than once a day, preferably only three to four times per week (see page 33).

Rye

Like wheat, rye contains gluten and is often best avoided in the early stages of treatment. It can often be reintroduced into the diet before wheat, in the form of crisp-breads, rye flakes and rye bread.

Barley

Barley also contains gluten but It tends to cause fewer problems than wheat and is likely only to be used in small quantities in dishes such as soups and casseroles. Avoid if you have gluten intolerance.

Oats

Although oats also contain gluten, they are generally more easily tolerated than wheat. Avoid oats if your health is seriously below par or if you have gluten intolerance. Otherwise include them no more than once per day.

Fruit

Limit yourself to one or two fruits per day. Avoid fruit juice or substitute one small glass of fruit juice for two pieces of fruit. Limit tropical fruits and very acidic fruits such as oranges, grapefruit, plums and strawberries. Apples and pears are the best fruit to be eaten regularly. Fruit may need to be avoided in the early stages of treating Candida albicans.

Dried Fruit

Use in moderation, preferably choosing unsulphurized. Avoid in the early stages of treating Candida albicans, if you have an intolerance to yeast, or suffer from flatulence or bloating. Washing dried fruit helps to remove some of the surface yeast.

Sugar

Avoid all sugar, brown or white. Avoid honey, molasses, malt extract and chemical sugar replacers.

Fats and Oils

Avoid or limit hardened fats and avoid hydrogenated margarine. For spreading, use low-salt butter, sparingly or a non-hydrogenated margarine (which is low in trans fatty acids). Use olive oil in any heated dishes, and sweat foods (see page 49) instead of frying, whenever possible. For salad dressings, olive oil is a good choice (see 'Fats and Oils', page 26).

Salt

Avoid salt completely for three to four months to allow your natural taste buds to develop. Use a potassium salt substitute if desired, and potassium baking powder in breads and cakes. Watch out for hidden forms of salt and sodium (see 'Salt', page 28).

Yeast

Avoid yeast, yeast extracts, shoyu/tamari/soya sauce, miso, vinegar, monosodium glutamate, citric acid, alcohol and stock cubes. Mushrooms and dried fruit may need to be excluded from the diet if you have yeast intolerance or Candida albicans is a problem (see 'Candida albicans', page 8).

Beverages

Avoid tea, coffee, carbonated soft drinks, squashes and alcohol (for advice on fruit juice, see page 33). Substitute with herb teas, rooibosch tea, coffee substitutes and filtered water. Look out for additives, such as lactose, gluten and flavourings, in alternative drinks. Be aware that it will take time for you to acquire a taste for alternatives. Also accept that you will miss tea and coffee – remember they are drugs. Persevere and make the change gradually.

Water

Try to drink at least 1.5 litres (3 pints/7½ cups) of bottled or filtered water per day (preferably warm or at room temperature) to assist detox-ification.

Tinned and Frozen Produce

Avoid the general use of tinned produce, but the occasional can of tuna, tomatoes and beans, for instance, is acceptable (choose those free from added sugar and salt). Limit frozen foods. Frozen fish and meat are allowed but use fresh vegetables for most meals. Frozen vegetables, such as sweetcorn or peas, used occasionally are acceptable as they help to make meals more interesting.

Additives

These include colourings, flavourings, preservatives, antioxidants, emulsifiers, stabilizers, sweeteners and modified starches. Addi-tives are mostly chemically derived and, as such, are another toxic substance for the body to deal with. Flavourings will often contain 100 chemicals just to produce one flavour. They have been shown to cause epileptic fits, asthma and hyperactivity, but often the underlying damage is unseen. Learn to read labels before you buy, but do be aware that some additives are naturally derived and are acceptable.

Suggested Menus

Breakfast

Rice porridge with cinnamon, cloves and dates. Millet porridge with fresh fruit, nuts and seeds. Soaked muesli with fresh fruit and soya milk. Egg fried rice. Scrambled eggs with cornmeal bread.

Mid-Morning

Eat a snack of rice served with fresh fruit and nuts, homemade soup or chopped vegetables. Alternatively, eat a second course for breakfast and have a piece of fresh fruit and some nuts mid-morning. Try fruit and nut or savoury rice slices (see recipes), they are easy to pick up and eat and are delicious.

Lunch

Eat a substantial lunch. Try homemade soup. Followed by a large mixed salad and a baked potato or a rice salad. If you prefer, try stir-fried vegetables with rice or a vegetarian savoury with salad.

Mid-Afternoon

Eat another snack; the size will depend on how late you eat your evening meal. Eat a bowl of rice with fruit and nuts or some rice slices. Rice cakes are delicious served with nut butter and mashed banana or sliced avocado and tomato or try some of the pâtés in the starter section (see page 69).

Evening Meal

A fish, chicken or vegetarian savoury served with a good selection of fresh vegetables and/or salad, plus a portion of rice, millet, buckwheat or quinoa and, occasionally, potatoes.

Supper

Try soup with rice, porridge, rice with fruit, rice slices, pear and carob delight, apple, date and nut muffins. If you tend to wake up feeling tired or if you are not usually hungry at breakfast-time, eating supper will help maintain your blood sugar levels overnight and enable you to eat a good breakfast. If you normally feel full of energy when you wake it is because your adrenal glands have had a rest; don't live on them, feed them!

Cooking Ingredients and Methods

Brown Rice

Some recipes call for cooked rice, others have quantities listed for uncooked rice. If you wish to substitute one for another you should note that rice approximately doubles in weight when cooked. If, there-fore, a recipe calls for 225g (8 oz/1 cup) of uncooked rice and you already have some cooked, then substitute 455g (16 oz/2½ cups). Rice will keep for two days if stored in the fridge or it can be frozen for those emergency situations. A Tupperware rice container is useful for both sieving and storing cooked rice. Most people find their own favourite way of cooking rice; here is mine.

COOKING BROWN RICE.
Soak 225g (8oz/1 cup) short-grain brown rice in a pan with lots of cold water for approximately 10 minutes. This loosens any dirt on the rice and prevents a scum forming when it is cooking. Strain the rice and place in a pan with 1¼ litres (2 pints/5 cups) of boiling water. Bring to the boil and simmer for 25–35 minutes. There will still be lots of water left in the pan. Strain the rice through a sieve and allow it to drain. Serve hot or leave to cool in the sieve, placed over the pan with the pan lid on top to prevent the rice from drying out. Long-grain brown rice does not take as long to cook as short-grain rice, but cooking times can vary with different batches of rice.

FLAVOURING BROWN RICE

Brown rice can be cooked in stock to add flavour. It can also be flavoured whilst cooking with herbs or spices (such as coriander, fennel or a bay leaf), or it can be cooked with the addition of onion, garlic or fresh ginger. Add more than one flavouring to produce interesting variations. Cooked rice can be flavoured by adding one or more of the following; toasted sunflower or sesame seeds, slivered almonds, grated orange or lemon rind, fresh herbs (coriander, mint, parsley), olive oil.

Millet, Buckwheat and Quinoa

These grains can be used in recipes as an alternative to boiled rice. To cook, follow the instructions for cooking brown rice, but cook buckwheat and quinoa for approximately 10 minutes and millet for approximately 18 minutes. Try using in nut roast, salads and rice slices. Like rice, millet doubles in weight once cooked. Buckwheat and quinoa treble in weight, so if substituting for rice in recipes, adjust accordingly.

Cooking Beans

Cooking time depends on the age of the beans (old beans take longer), the size of the beans and the length of the soaking time. Smaller beans and pulses, such as lentils, mung beans, aduki beans and split peas, can be cooked without soaking. Larger beans need soaking overnight in plenty of cold water. Discard the soaking water and rinse well before cooking. Because some beans contain toxins, it is best to fast boil all beans for the first ten minutes to render the toxins harmless. Even after soaking, large beans can take up to two hours to cook. This is where I find a pressure cooker invaluable as most large beans can be cooked in only five minutes after an overnight soak. They are not mushy at this stage but are ready to place in dishes such as casseroles and soups. Beans approximately double in size when soaked and cooked.

Beans can be frozen at the soaked stage or at the just-cooked stage so that a supply is always at hand. Try freezing them in a colander or sieve as this allows excess water to drain away. The beans can then be tipped into a plastic bag where, with a little encouragement, they will become free flowing, allowing you to take out just the amount you need at any time.

I always keep a few tins of beans in the cupboard for those emergency situations. Some do, however, contain salt so I discard the liquid and rinse well. Tinned beans do seem to be easier to digest and appear to cause less flatulence than the dried variety.

Stock

Stock can be made from leftover bones, fresh bones, giblets, vegetables and vegetable cooking water. Stock is also becoming increasingly available, ready prepared, from the supermarkets. Vegetables should always be steamed or cooked in as little water as possible to prevent minerals leaching into the cooking water. However, saving any leftover cooking liquid for soup stock will add flavour and minerals to the soup. I keep a container in the ice box of my fridge, and each day add any leftover cooking water to it. When I am ready to make soup the stock is ready. Do not use stock from cauliflower or other strong-tasting vegetables, as this will alter the flavour of the soup.

Bones can be obtained from most butchers, but do not use bacon bones as these contain sodium. Raw bones produce better flavoured stock if they are roasted first in a hot oven until brown. Stock made from bones should be brought to the boil and simmered for an hour, making sure that the water level just covers the bones. A pressure cooker saves time when making stock. When cooked, strain the stock, allow to cool, then remove any fat from the surface. Try to cook stock in large quantities and freeze some so that stock is always available.

For fish stock ask your fishmonger for bones and boil these in sufficient water to cover them for just 10 minutes. Cooking longer gives the stock a strong, bitter flavour.

Sprouted Seeds

Sprouting seeds can be grown from most whole beans and pulses, but your supply needs to be fresh, as old seeds do not sprout well. Some of the easiest to grow are lentils, alfalfa, mung and aduki. You can buy special trays for growing seeds, but a jam jar will suffice.

Place 15 ml (1 tbsp) of the seeds in the jar and soak overnight in lots of cold water. The following morning, either fasten a piece of muslin over the jam jar or use the lid to strain the water from the seeds. Rinse the seeds in more fresh water then drain again, and this time leave to stand in a warm, preferably dark, place (a dark jar can be used). Each morning and evening, rinse and drain the jar. In two to three days (depending on the warmth), you will have sprouts ready to eat. They are ready when leaves begin to appear.

Freezing Orange and Lemon – Juice and Rind

These should not be used in large quantities as they cause excess elimination of toxins from the cells, which, if not removed by the body, can cause symptoms to appear. They are, however, ideal used in small quantities to add flavour to recipes. I keep ice cubes made from orange and lemon juice in the freezer for such occasions. Orange and lemon rind can also be frozen, but preferably buy organically grown fruit as most fruits will have been heavily sprayed. Grate and loosely pack into small containers. If you cannot tolerate citrus fruits, leave these flavourings out of recipes.

Freezing Ginger

Fresh ginger goes mouldy quite quickly even if kept in the fridge, so peel a large piece of ginger and freeze. Whenever you need ginger for a recipe, grate a little whilst it is still frozen and return the rest to the freezer. It is surprisingly easy to grate.

Freezing Herbs

I like to use fresh herbs whenever possible but I also like to freeze herbs so that a supply is always available. I grow or buy herbs, chop them and place in small containers in the freezer. If you do not have fresh or frozen herbs, substitute dried herbs, but use only one quarter of the fresh amount.

Miso

Although miso is a fermented soya product containing salt, it is such a good food nutritionally that it is worth including in the diet if it can be tolerated. If you have Candida albicans or yeast intolerance, you will need to avoid miso for a long period and should use it sparingly when it is eventually introduced. The salt content of miso is approximately 8–10 per cent. Some miso contains barley or wheat, so check the ingredients. Use miso in the same way as you would stock cubes by dissolving in a small amount of boiling water.

Shoyu/Tamari/Soya Sauce

These sauces are made from fermented soya beans which produce a deep, rich flavour that tastes saltier than it is. Shoyu and tamari are both available from health-food shops. Soya sauce is available from supermarkets but usually contains wheat and monosodium glutamate. Avoid tamari, shoyu and soya sauce if you have Candida albicans or yeast intolerance.

Seaweeds

Although seaweed does contain salt, wash well and use in soups, casseroles and salads, as seaweed is a very good natural source of vitamins and minerals.

Mustard

Mustard usually has added vinegar or wheat, but you can find mustard flour with no other added ingredients and English mustard with only salt added (see 'Useful Addresses', page 260).

Vinegar Substitutes

Use the equivalent amount of lemon juice or try powdered vitamin C instead of vinegar – 2ml (¼ tsp) for each 15 ml (1 tbsp) of vinegar.

Olives

Most olives seem to be preserved in brine, but you can buy olives in olive oil from some delicatessens. Some contain other additives, such as citric acid, which needs to be avoided. Because olives are used only in small quantities and give a wonderful flavour to dishes, I accept the small amount of additional salt.

Tomatoes

If you cannot tolerate tomatoes but can use miso or tamari, then use these in recipes instead of tomato puree. Where a tin or carton of tomato juice is listed in the ingredients, substitute carrot or other vegetable juices.

Sun-Dried Tomatoes

These are available bottled in olive oil although many do seem to contain vinegar or citric acid (check labels). I have, however, found sun-dried tomatoes in a packet with no additives. These need soaking in water to soften.

Pasta

Delicious forms of pasta are now being made from ingredients such as rice, cornmeal, millet, buckwheat and vegetables instead of wheat.

Egg Replacers

Egg replacers can be used to bind ingredients together but will not help a mixture to rise. These are readily available in health-food shops. Alternatively, an egg replacer can be made by simmering together for five minutes 15 ml (1 tbsp) of flax seeds and 115 ml (4 fl oz/½ cup) of water. This will produce a mixture which is the consistency of raw egg white and equates to one egg. You do not need to strain the mixture, as the seeds will just add flavour to your recipe.

Puffed Rice Cakes

These are often used as a snack food or a substitute for bread. There is no problem with this except that rice cakes contain mainly air and very little rice. Only use them to accompany a substantial meal or snack.

Thickeners

Corn flour has been used as a thickening agent in some recipes. Other flours can be substituted but the amount used may need to be adjusted. To thicken 425 ml (¾ pint/2 cups) of liquid use one of the following:

15 ml (1 level tbsp) potato flour
30 ml (2 level tbsp) rice flour or corn flour
45 ml (3 level tbsp) gram flour, soya flour or polenta flour

Raising Agents

Most baking powders contain ingredients such as aluminium and wheat, as well as being sodium based. Health food shops sell sodium baking powders free from gluten and aluminium but potassium baking powder free from gluten and additives is more acceptable. This is becoming more readily available, so ask in your local health food shop, or see the 'List of Suppliers' on page 259.

Stevia

Stevia is an alternative sweetener. Extracts of stevia, a South American shrub, are estimated to be up to 300 times sweeter than sugar but stevia has no calories. The herb has been shown to be non-toxic and safe for diabetics and hypoglycaemics. In addition, stevia does not nourish the bacteria in the mouth, as sugars do, nor does it stimulate the growth of Candida in the digestive tract. (See 'List of Suppliers' page 259).

Food Families

Individuals with severe allergies or food intolerance may find that foods related to the ones to which they are intolerant can also cause problems. Ignore the list below unless you are still having trouble with your diet after a few months, in which case it may be worth avoiding the foods related to your problem foods.

Banana	ginger, tumeric, cardamom.
Beet	chard, spinach, sugar (beet), beetroot.
Carrot	caraway, celery, chervil, coriander, cumin, dill, fennel, parsley, parsnip, celeriac.
Cashew	mango, pistachio.
Compositae	lettuce, chicory, sunflower, safflower, dandelion, camomile, artichoke.
Grasses	wheat, corn, barley, oats, millet, cane sugar, bamboo shoots, rice, rye (buckwheat is not a member of the grass family).
Legume	beans, lentils, liquorice, peas, senna, soya, string beans.
Mustard	broccoli, Brussels sprouts, cabbage, Chinese leaves, cauliflower, cress, horseradish, kale, kohlrabi, radish, swede, turnip, watercress, rapeseed.
Palm	coconut, date, sago.
Potato	aubergine, pepper, chilli, tobacco, tomato, cape gooseberry.
Rose	apple, pear, apricot, cherry, peach, plum, blackberry, raspberry, strawberry.

Putting Cooking Without Into Practice

When you start following this eating regime, I suggest that you eat six meals per day. This enables the body to obtain energy from food rather than through the release of adrenalin or from the liver's glycogen stores. The energy that comes from eating regularly will not only make you feel better but will also enable the internal organs and systems of the body to recover and remove any toxic build-up.

Food may initially have to be forced into the body at regular intervals, as individuals with low blood sugar do not always feel like eating and can even feel sick at the thought of food. Once the blood sugar has been raised by the intake of food, however, the body seems grateful and will actually start asking to be fed at regular intervals. During this phase you need to make sure that you always have a snack with you wherever you are going in order to keep topping up the blood sugar. Miss the snack and let the blood sugar fall and you will spend the rest of the day feeling under par, chasing your blood sugar but never actually catching it up.

Eventually, when the body has removed excess toxins and obtained sufficient vitamins and minerals from the improved diet, three meals per day should be adequate, with an occasional piece of fruit in between. By then the liver should be supporting the blood sugar between meals, and adrenalin can be kept for emergency situations. Your body will tell you when you are ready for this; it may be in three months' time or it may be in two years' time, depending on the state of your health when you start detoxifying. Suddenly, you will find that you do not feel hungry all the time, and you will happily last from one meal to the next.

Organizing Your Cooking

Do not think that *Cooking Without* is about denying food. See it rather as about building health – eating the right kind of food in sufficient quantities at regular intervals.

Health is like a bank balance – when we become ill we have gone into the red. Even though we are overdrawn, we still have to spend energy just to do the bare essentials each day. In order to obtain health we need to minimize the amount of energy spent whilst at the same time putting as much as possible back into the bank by feeding ourselves as well as we can. In this way we eventually return our health balance to the black and have a few reserves in store for a rainy day.

It only takes a change in attitude to put food and feeding ourselves correctly at the top of our priority list for the day, rather than at the bottom, where it fits in if there is any time left. We would not dream of jumping into the car and covering up the warning light because it was indicating that the petrol tank was empty, yet how often do we do this with our bodies? By feeding ourselves well today and every day we will have many more years when we can work, look after our families, help others, play sport and live our lives well. If we do not put the effort in now, we will run out of reserves sooner or later and become ill.

Try to organize your cooking so that you have lots of tempting dishes available when you open the fridge door. In this way you will not think about what you cannot eat but rather about what you can enjoy. Put aside a few hours once or twice a week to make quite a few dishes at the same time. If you are chopping vegetables for a casserole, you might as well chop some for soup and a terrine at the same time. You could bake fruit and nut slices whilst preparing a nut roast and corn-meal bread.

When cooked, decant some of the food into the freezer for emergency situations or for use later in the week. I like to place a few individual portions in 'au gratin' dishes in the freezer, but you could just fill containers with larger amounts. The rest of the food can be kept in the fridge so that for the next few days you have plenty to tempt you. If you always keep some brown rice cooked (it will keep for up to two days in the fridge), you only need to rustle up a salad or cook some fresh vegetables to complete a meal.

If family members do not want to change their eating patterns to fit in with you, then try making lots of dishes as suggested above, plus a few which they like. Spread the dishes out on the table for a buffet meal, but without making a distinction between their food and yours. Eventually, they will start to accept the new regime.

Make the Change Gradually

It is a good idea to start the new regime gradually, perhaps over a period of one to four weeks, depending on how good your diet is to start with. The body is used to coping with foods such as meat, wheat, tea and coffee, which suppress the elimination of toxins and push them back into the cells. By removing or reducing such foods and increasing the amount of vegetables eaten, toxins are encouraged to flow out of the cells. If, however, they flow out of the cells faster than the body can eliminate them to the outside world, excess toxins float around in the bloodstream, making you feel worse rather than better. This may cause a headache, anxiety, tiredness, an upset stomach or can aggravate symptoms already present. If you feel any adverse reactions to the diet then make the change more gradual, but do not give up. Your body is probably saying, 'Thank goodness! At last I can get rid of this toxic, acid waste.'

We are so used to ignoring our bodies and panicking when symptoms appear that it takes time to gain an understanding of how the body works and what it is saying. As you gain health, you will also gain confidence in your body and will no longer fear growing old and becoming ill.

Widening the Range of Foods Consumed

The length of time for which this dietary regime needs to be adhered to will depend on the severity of your health problems. You may need to follow the diet for anything from a few months to a few years. Once your health has improved, try widening the range of foods consumed, but be prepared to go back to the strict regime if you do not feel as well. When reintroducing foods, try one new food at a time to see how it affects you.

You should eventually be able to reintroduce wheat, rye, barley and oats, but I recommend that you do not include wheat more than once per day. A little milk in your barleycup or rooibosch tea is acceptable, and cottage cheese and yogurt can be eaten occasionally. Salt is needed only in the occasional soup or casserole. Miso and shoyu or tamari sauce are ideal for flavouring soups and casseroles as they have many beneficial properties. A little cider vinegar, honey, molasses and sugar-free fruit spreads can be used in moderation.

The benefits you receive from *Cooking Without,* will, I hope, encourage you to make this way of eating the foundation on which to build your own individual diet for life.

Weight Control

Do not worry about putting on excess weight by eating more food more often. Provided that you are only eating the foods suggested in this book, then everything in the body will function more efficiently, including the metabolism. The art of weight control is to keep the blood sugar supported. The result will be a weight loss for those who are carrying any excess. Anyone who is underweight will need to eat heartily on this regime as it does not encourage weight gain. However, underweight people often live on nervous energy, which burns up calories. Because *Cooking Without* affects mental and emotional states, it promotes relaxation which in turn lessens the use of nervous energy. This has the effect of encouraging weight gain where this is the cause.

Vegetarians

This diet is ideally suited to vegetarians. Non-vegetarian ingredients included in some recipes are optional. Omitting them will speed up the elimination process still further. If you have suddenly decided to become vegetarian, then I suggest that you change over gradually to avoid excess elimination of toxins and to allow your body to become accustomed to the change.

Vitamin and Mineral Supplements

Nutritional supplements, especially minerals, assist the elimination of toxins from the body. It is, however, impossible in a book such as this to suggest levels suitable for all readers. If you wish to use supplements to assist the detoxification process, consult a qualified nutritional therapist (see 'Useful Addresses', page 260).

Equipment

Do not cook with aluminium pans, as aluminium is a toxic metal. Non-stick pans have similar problems. Pressure cookers are usually made of aluminium, but are available in stainless steel.

A food processor is a labour-saving piece of equipment. It can be used for slicing, chopping or shredding vegetables and it will also liquidize, purée and mix. If a food processor is not available, then in many instances, a liquidizer or blender can be used.

When cup measurements only are given (in breakfast recipes), I use a tea cup but the size does not matter as long as you keep the proportions the same. Cup measurements in other recipes refer to American cup measures.

General Information

I have tried to include alternative ingredients in many instances, but this is not always possible without making recipes excessively long. Most recipes, however, will adapt to substitutions. Vegetables can be exchanged in recipes, and alternative flours can be used in baking. Egg substitutes can be used in most recipes, and nut or rice milk can be used instead of soya milk. Ingredients used to add flavour, such as tomato purée, orange juice or lemon rind, can be omitted.

Sweating is used in quite a few recipes to impart more flavour. This is not the same as frying as you cook at a lower temperature. It involves softening the vegetables in oil, at a low temperature in an uncovered pan. The vegetables need to be stirred regularly with a wooden spoon until they begin to cook and brown. Sweating does take time. Allow at least 20 minutes, and sweat vegetables whilst you collect other ingredients together to save time.

Folding is used in a few recipes and involves mixing ingredients using a metal spoon and following a figure-of-eight movement. This prevents the air being beaten out of the ingredients.

I have tried to keep oven temperatures the same in many recipes so that you can bake several dishes at the same time.

BreakfastBreakfastBreakfastBreakfast

Breakfast is a very important meal. First thing in the morning, we are literally breaking our night's fast. If you have difficulty eating breakfast or feel sick at the thought of it, this means that your blood sugar has dropped too low overnight. Start by eating small amounts of breakfast, perhaps fruit or something light to start with, and gradually increase this amount until a substantial breakfast is not only acceptable, but actually desired.

It is occasionally necessary for some people to eat in the middle of the night to prevent the blood sugar dropping so low. When toxicity has eventually been removed and sufficient minerals have been obtained, blood sugar levels will be stable for longer periods. If the blood sugar is not raised by eating breakfast first thing in the morning, then people often spend all day chasing it but never achieving stability or feeling good, however much they eat.

If you like to lie in at the weekend, take your breakfast to bed with you. Set the alarm as normal, eat your breakfast and go back to sleep making sure that you are up before your mid-morning snack. If you normally feel worse after a lie-in, it is because your blood sugar levels have dropped too low by the time you eat.

Although I have tried to make the recipes in this section conform to typical breakfast dishes, what you eat for breakfast does not really matter as long as it raises your blood sugar. Some breakfast dishes could be used for meals and snacks during the day, such as Bubble and Squeak for lunch or Pear and Carob Delight as a pudding or supper dish. Other breakfast suggestions include breads from Chapter 9, Rice Pudding (see page 240), Kedgeree (see page 191) and eggs, boiled, scrambled or poached.

As all the recipes are gluten-free, they exclude oats, a delicious breakfast cereal. I have noted where oats can be substituted for those who do not have a problem with gluten. Millet flakes have a distinctive flavour which takes some adjusting to, as do buckwheat flakes which can be used instead of, or as well as, millet flakes.

If dried fruit cannot be tolerated because of Candida albicans or yeast intolerance, then omit it from these recipes and use fresh fruit in its place. Some may be able to tolerate crystallized pineapple and ginger or dried apple better than dried fruit. Although ginger and pineapple do contain some sugar, the amounts are small and they may help to make a dish more agreeable to some people.

Muesli

Oat flakes can be substituted for the millet flakes if gluten can be tolerated. Vary the fruit and nuts so that each muesli you make is different, for example, hazelnut and apricot, raisin and almond or mixed fruit and nut. If you cannot tolerate dried fruit, serve the muesli with fresh fruit, either raw or stewed.

7 cups millet flakes	1 cup coconut flakes *or* ¼ cup
½ cup sunflower seeds	desiccated coconut
1 cup nuts	1 cup dried fruit (optional)

1 Mix all the ingredients together and store in a container.
2 Serve with soya, almond or rice milk and fresh fruit.

Light Muesli

Oats can be substituted for the millet flakes if gluten can be tolerated. Serve with fresh fruit if dried fruit is not allowed.

4 cups puffed rice cereal	¾ cup mixed dried fruit e.g.
¾ cup mixed nuts	chopped dates, apricots, figs,
½ cup sunflower seeds	raisins *or* sultanas (optional)
4 cups millet flakes	½ cup desiccated coconut

1 Mix all the ingredients together and store in a container.
2 Serve with soya, almond or rice milk.

Millet Porridge

Oat porridge can be made in the same way for those who can tolerate oats.

INGREDIENTS PER PERSON: | 2¾ cups cold water
1 cup millet flakes |

1 Place the ingredients in a pan and bring to the boil, stirring.
2 Simmer gently for approximately 10 minutes.
3 Serve plain with soya, almond or rice milk or with fresh fruit, dried fruit, nuts and seeds piled on top. These could be added to the porridge whilst it is cooking to vary the recipe.

Soaked Muesli

This muesli is ideal to take on holiday as it can be easily made up in hotel bedrooms and can also be used for between-meal snacks. My favourite version of this recipe contains 55g/2 oz/½ cup of crystallized pineapple instead of 55g/2 oz/½ cup of the raisins, and I use whole almonds for the nuts. Oats can be substituted for the millet flakes if gluten is allowed. Serve with fresh fruit if dried fruit is not tolerated.

340g/12 oz/3 cups rice flakes | 255g/9 oz/3 cups millet flakes
115g/4 oz/1 cup raisins *or* | 55g/2 oz/½ cup sunflower seeds
mixed dried fruit (optional) | 55g/2 oz/½ cup nuts

1 Mix all the ingredients together and store in an airtight container.
2 Fill a breakfast bowl with the muesli and soak in sufficient water just to cover the ingredients. Allow to stand for at least 15 minutes or, if desired, soak overnight.
3 Serve with soya, almond or rice milk, soya yogurt or just as it is.

Rice Porridge

Rice flakes vary a lot in the amount of water they soak up, so adjust the liquid if necessary.

INGREDIENTS PER PERSON:
170g/6 oz/1 cup brown rice flakes
2ml/¼ tsp cinnamon
1ml/⅛ tsp ground cloves
570ml/20 fl oz/2½ cups boiling water

10ml/1 dsp dried fruit e.g. raisins, dates (optional)
½ piece fresh fruit e.g. apple, pear, banana

1 Place all the ingredients except the fresh fruit into a pan, bring to the boil and simmer gently for 10 minutes, stirring occasionally.
2 Cut the fresh fruit into pieces and add to the pan 2 minutes before the end of cooking or pile on top just before serving.

Breakfast Rice

1 bowl of cooked rice per person plus a selection from the following:

- nuts and seeds
- spices e.g. nutmeg, cinnamon
- finely diced dried fruit
- chopped fresh fruit
- carob powder
- desiccated coconut
- soya milk, rice milk, fruit juice *or* soya yogurt
- stewed fresh fruit
- stewed dried fruit

It is a good idea to keep toppings such as nuts, seeds, toasted nuts and seeds and chopped dried fruit in clear glass jars on your work surface or shelf. Then you can quickly add toppings to a bowl of warm or cold rice. Children love the idea of helping themselves to toppings.

Suggested combinations for 1 bowl of rice:

- ½ chopped banana, a few cashew nuts *or* raisins.
- ½ stewed apple, pinch cinnamon, toasted sunflower seeds.
- ½ pear, chopped dried apricots, toasted slivered almonds.
- Liquidize ½ peach and ½ banana and pour over the rice.
- Stewed prunes and soya yogurt.
- Stewed dried apricots and chopped almonds.
- ½ pear, nutmeg and warm soya milk.
- 5ml/1tsp carob flour, pinch nutmeg and warm soya milk.

Pear and Carob Delight

A banana can be substituted for the pear in this recipe.

INGREDIENTS PER PERSON:
40ml/2 rounded tbsp rice flour
10ml/1 dsp carob flour
170ml/6 fl oz/¾ cup soya *or*
almond milk

1 small pear
10ml/1 dsp desiccated coconut
170ml/6 fl oz/¾ cup boiling
water

1 In a pan mix the rice and carob flour to a smooth paste with a little milk. Gradually add the remaining milk.
2 Cut the pear into thin slices and add to the pan with the coconut.
3 Add the boiling water and bring the mixture to the boil, stirring.
4 Lower the heat and simmer for 5–10 minutes or until the pear begins to disintegrate, sweetening the mixture.

Banana and Maize Breakfast Cereal

If desired, a piece of vanilla pod can be used instead of the extract, and a pear can be substituted for the banana.

INGREDIENTS PER PERSON:
40ml/2 rounded tbsp cornflour
170ml/6 fl oz/¾ cup soya *or*
almond milk

2 drops natural vanilla extract
170ml/6 fl oz/¾ cup boiling
water
1 small banana

1 Mix the cornflour to a smooth paste with the milk in a pan.
2 Add the vanilla extract, the boiling water and the finely sliced banana.
3 Bring the mixture to the boil, stirring constantly.
4 Lower the heat and simmer for 5–10 minutes or until the banana begins to disintegrate.

Sago Breakfast Cereal

If desired, a piece of vanilla pod can be used instead of the extract. Sago does seem to vary in the amount of liquid it absorbs. Adjust the recipe if necessary.

INGREDIENTS PER PERSON:
40ml/2 rounded tbsp sago
½ banana or pear, chopped
200ml/7 fl oz/¾ cup soya or almond milk

2 drops natural vanilla extract
200ml/7 fl oz/¾ cup boiling water
10ml/1 dsp finely chopped dates (optional)

1 Place all the ingredients into a pan, bring to the boil, stirring constantly, then lower the heat.
2 Simmer for 15–20 minutes, stirring occasionally.
3 The fruit should begin to disintegrate, sweetening the mixture.

Soya Milk Yogurt

The mixture ideally needs to fill a flask in order for the yogurt to stay warm. Adjust the quantities if your flask is larger.

Yogurt culture can be bought to use as a starter or use 5ml/1 tsp of a bought soya yogurt. Even though these normally contain some sugar there will be very little in the amount used. The yogurt will not take as long to set if using soya yogurt or a culture instead of the acidophilus.

570ml/1 pint/2½ cups organic soya milk

4 milk-free acidophilus capsules

1 Bring the milk to the boil and then allow to cool to body temperature (a clean finger is sufficient to test). Cover the pan to prevent a skin forming.

2 Empty the acidophilus capsules into a small basin and add 1 tsp of the warm soya milk, mixing until you have a smooth paste. Continue adding the soya milk and mixing until the acidophilus is well blended, then pour into the pan and stir.
3 Pour the mixture into a warmed vacuum flask, put the top on and leave to stand for approximately 6 hours or until the mixture just starts to leave the sides of the flask when the flask is tipped.
4 Tip the yogurt out into a container and store in the fridge.

Almond Milk

Other nuts, such as cashews, can be used instead of almonds. The milk will keep for 48 hours in the fridge but will separate a little on standing. Shake before using.

½ cup blanched almonds	485ml/17 fl oz/2¼ cups water

1 To blanch the almonds, pour boiling water over the nuts and leave them to stand for 5 minutes. The skins should then easily slip off when pressed with the thumb.
2 Place the nuts in a blender and blend until finely ground.
3 Add 125ml/4 fl oz/½ cup of water and blend until a smooth cream is formed.
4 Add the remaining water and blend well.
5 Put the mixture through a fine sieve. If there is a great deal of pulp left, you have not blended for long enough.

Breakfast in a Glass

Try substituting other fresh fruits such as peaches, apricots and mango, or add 5ml/1 tsp carob powder to the banana.

1 banana *or* other soft fruit 40ml/2 heaped tbsp cooked rice pinch nutmeg	90ml/3 fl oz/⅓ cup soya, almond *or* rice milk

1 Place all the ingredients in a food processor and liquidize until smooth.
2 Pour the mixture into a glass and eat as you would a yogurt.

Marmalade

2 oranges (preferably organic) *or* 1 orange and 1 lemon	225g/8 oz/1¼ cups dried apricots, cut into pieces 140ml/5 fl oz/⅔ cup water

1 Wash the oranges well and squeeze the juice from them.
2 Place the juice in a pan along with the apricot pieces.
3 Bring the apricots and juice to the boil, lower the heat, place a lid on the pan and simmer for approximately 10 minutes or until the apricots are soft. Add a little water if the mixture starts to become too dry. The amount of water needed and the length of cooking time will be determined by how old the apricots are.
4 Cut the peel from the oranges into matchstick-size pieces and place in a pan along with the water.
5 Bring to the boil and simmer for 10 minutes or until the peel is soft.
6 Process the apricots and juice to form a soft, smooth purée.
7 Mix together the apricot purée, the orange peel and any juices from the pan. Add a little more liquid if the mixture is too stiff.
8 Allow to cool. Place the marmalade into two jars or containers.

I suggest you store one in the fridge where it will keep for up to two weeks and the other in the freezer.

Fruit Spread

Fruit spreads can be made by stewing and liquidizing fresh or dried fruit. Do not include the cooking liquid as this will make the spread too runny. If the spread is still too soft, thicken with a little arrowroot or Gelozone (the vegetarian equivalent of gelatine, available in health-food shops and some supermarkets). Try apple and cinnamon, dried apricot or mixed summer fruits. The spreads will not keep for more than a few days if made with fresh fruit.

Egg Fried Rice

Serves 4

15ml/1 tbsp of shoyu/tamari sauce will add extra flavour (if your diet allows). Try serving with a salad for lunch.

4 eggs	455g/1 lb/2½ cups cooked rice
80ml/8 dsp water	black pepper
10ml/1dsp olive oil	

1 Beat the eggs with 4 dsp water.
2 Pour 5ml/1 tsp of oil into a frying pan, heat and add the eggs. Cook as an omelette by lifting the edges of the mixture as it cooks and allowing any uncooked mixture to run to the base.
3 Cut the omelette into little pieces either in the pan or by removing and cutting on a chopping board.
4 Place the cooked egg and rice into the pan along with 5ml/1 tsp of oil and the black pepper. Stir-fry until heated through.
5 Add the remaining 4 dsp water and allow this to be absorbed, then serve.

Scrambled Tofu with Sweetcorn and Arame

Serves 4

Use 10ml/1 dsp of water in the pan if you prefer not to fry. 10ml/1 dsp of shoyu/tamari sauce can be added (if your diet allows).

80ml/4tbsp arame seaweed	225g/8 oz/2 cups tofu, plain *or*
5ml/1 tsp olive oil	smoked
225g/8 oz/1¼ cups sweetcorn kernels	

1 Soak the arame in boiling water for approximately 10 minutes or until soft. Sieve to remove the water.
2 Place the olive oil in a pan then add the arame, the sweetcorn and the tofu crumbled into tiny pieces.
3 Warm through by stir-frying, and serve.

Rice with Leeks and Scrambled Eggs

Serves 4

455g/1 lb/4 cups leeks, chopped	6 eggs
455g/1 lb/2½ cups cooked rice	black pepper

1 Cook the leeks in a little water until just tender. Drain well.
2 Warm the rice if not freshly cooked.
3 Beat the eggs with 45ml/3 tbsp of water and scramble.
4 Mix all the ingredients together and season with black pepper.

Potato Cakes

Serves 4

Try substituting parsnips for the potatoes if these cause a problem.

680g/1½ lb/5 cups potatoes	15ml/1 tbsp olive oil
60ml/3 rounded tbsp rice flour	extra flour for shaping
black pepper	

1 Peel, chop and cook the potatoes in boiling water until soft.
2 Sieve and keep the liquid. Mash the potatoes until smooth using a little of the cooking liquid or soya milk to moisten.
3 Add the rice flour and pepper and mix well.
4 Take handfuls of the mixture and roll into balls using rice flour to keep the mixture from sticking to your hands. Flatten the balls into cakes approximately 1½ cm/½ inch thick.
5 Fry the cakes in a little oil until they begin to brown (approximately 5 minutes). Turn and fry the other side. Serve spread with butter if allowed or to accompany other breakfast dishes.

Traditional English Breakfast

Serves 4

Try to buy organic kidneys or liver and soak overnight in a little soya milk if you prefer a less strong flavour. Baked beans bought from a health-food shop may be acceptable but check the ingredients first.

4 whole kidneys *or* 4 pieces lamb's liver olive oil and black pepper 4 beef tomatoes	4–8 potato cakes 340g/12 oz/3 cups mushrooms 4 eggs

1 Cut the kidneys in half, skin them and remove the core. Brush the kidneys or liver with oil and sprinkle with black pepper. Grill for approximately 5 minutes on each side under a medium heat until they are cooked.
2 Cut the tomatoes in half, sprinkle with black pepper and place under the grill with the kidneys 2 minutes before the end of cooking. Warm the potato cakes in a similar way.
3 Clean and chop the mushrooms and fry in a little oil until just cooked.
4 Scramble or poach the eggs according to your preference.
5 Assemble the ingredients on 4 warm plates.

Sweetcorn and Onion Fritters

Serves 4

Try substituting other vegetables and beans in this recipe, such as peas and white cabbage or butterbeans and green peppers.

1 large onion, finely chopped	1 large egg, beaten
115g/4 oz/⅔ cup sweetcorn kernels	15ml/1 tbsp fresh parsley
70g/2½ oz/⅓ cup rice flour	black pepper
285ml/10 fl oz/1⅓ cups water	olive oil

1 Cook the onion in 30ml/2 tbsp water until soft. Drain.
2 Place the sweetcorn kernels in a bowl and roughly mash with the back of a fork until the kernels are just broken.
3 Add the onion, rice flour, water, egg, parsley and black pepper to the sweetcorn. Mix well.
4 Fry as two large pancakes in the olive oil until the pancakes are set and golden brown, turning half-way through cooking *(see the 'Bubble and Squeak' recipe on the next page for how to turn).*

Bubble and Squeak

Serves 4

Ideally, make this dish with leftover potatoes and cabbage for a quick breakfast dish. Other leftover vegetables could be substituted for the cabbage (such as carrots, peas and beans) and parsnips could be substituted for the potatoes if these cause problems.

680g/1½ lb/5 cups potatoes	black pepper
225g/8 oz/4 cups white cabbage	15ml/1 tbsp olive oil

1 Cook the potatoes in boiling water until soft.
2 Chop and cook the cabbage, preferably steamed over the potatoes. Do not over-cook.
3 Mash the potatoes with a little of the cooking water until soft and smooth. Add the cabbage and pepper and mix well.
4 Grease a frying pan with half of the olive oil and fry the potato mixture flattened into a pancake shape for approximately 10 minutes or until crisp and brown.
5 Slide the mixture out of the pan onto a chopping board, cooked side downwards. Grease the pan with the remaining oil and invert the pan over the potato mixture. Lift both the pan and the chopping board and turn over so that the mixture tips into the frying pan with the uncooked side downwards.
6 Cook for a further 10 minutes or until the second side is brown.

Potato Pancakes

Serves 2–4

1 egg, beaten	1 small onion, grated
55g/2 oz/⅓ cup rice flour	10ml/1 dsp chopped fresh
140ml/5 fl oz/⅔ cup water	parsley *or* other fresh herbs
255g/9 oz/2 cups grated raw	15ml/1 tbsp olive oil
potato	

1 Mix all the ingredients together, except the oil.
2 Fry as one large pancake in half of the oil for approximately 15 minutes, turning the heat down low after the first few minutes to prevent burning. Turn the pancake and fry in the remaining oil for a further 15 minutes. The outside of the pancake should be crisp and golden and the potatoes cooked through on the inside.

StartersStartersStartersStartersStar

ersStartersStartersStarters $\boxed{\text{Starters}}$

Starters can be used as snacks, light lunches or suppers. If you normally have a two-course evening meal involving a pudding, try serving a starter instead so that you avoid the pudding trap. Puddings can then be saved for weekends.

Many of the salads in Chapter 4 can be served as starters. Try minted avocado and chickpeas or curried egg and rice served on a bed of lettuce. If you do not like main-course salads, then serve a salad starter to benefit from eating more raw vegetables.

Stuffed Lettuce Leaves

Serves 4

Those allowed could use cottage cheese instead of tofu and serve with crusty bread to mop up the juices. Prawns contain salt unless freshly boiled. Avocado can be substituted for the eggs.

	STUFFING:
8 large soft lettuce leaves	2 hardboiled eggs
French dressing to serve *(see Chapter 8, page 198)*	15ml/1 tbsp fresh herbs e.g. parsley, mint, chives
cress to garnish	55g/2 oz/½ cup prawns
	40ml/2 tbsp grated tofu
	40ml/2 tbsp mayonnaise *(see page 200)*
	15g/½ oz/⅛ cup ground almonds
	2 ml/¼ tsp grated lemon rind

1 Finely chop the eggs and the herbs, then mix all the stuffing ingredients together.
2 Divide the stuffing mixture between the eight lettuce leaves, roll up and place two leaves on each plate.
3 Garnish with the cress and serve with French dressing.

VARIATIONS

Lettuce leaves can be stuffed with a selection of finely chopped or grated vegetables mixed with sufficient mayonnaise or yogurt to bind, such as avocado, tomato, pepper, spring onions (scallions), carrot, cucumber, sweetcorn, sprouted seeds. Some brown rice could be included.

Spinach and Carrot Timbale

Serves 4–6

This is a delicious dish to serve as a vegetarian main course along with Fresh Tomato Sauce *(see Chapter 8, page 204)*. Other vegetables could be substituted, such as parsnips for the carrots, and leeks or cauliflower instead of the spinach.

455g/1 lb/8 cups spinach	1 egg
455g/1 lb/3 cups carrots	1 clove garlic
2 ml/¼ tsp nutmeg	sliced tomato and toasted
black pepper	sesame seeds to garnish

1 Cook the spinach (in the water which remains on the leaves after washing) for no more than 5 minutes. Drain.
2 Cut the carrots into even-sized pieces and cook until just tender.
3 Purée the carrots with a little of the cooking liquid, the nutmeg and some black pepper.
4 Process the spinach with the egg, the garlic and lots of black pepper until a smooth purée is formed.
5 Place a layer of carrot purée, then a layer of spinach purée, into 4 gratin or 6 ramekin dishes.
6 Cover with foil and bake at 400°F/200°C/Gas Mark 6 for 10–15 minutes or until the spinach purée has set.
7 Garnish with sliced tomatoes and toasted sesame seeds.

Warm Chicken Liver Salad

Serves 4

Use coarse-grain mustard and organic chicken livers if possible. If allowed, add a knob of butter to the oil and mop up the juices with some crusty bread.

115g/4 oz/1⅓ cups continental salad leaves e.g. frisee, radicchio, lamb's lettuce (corn salad)	2 cloves garlic 225g/8 oz/1 cup chicken livers 10ml/1 dsp olive oil 5ml/1 tsp mustard

1 Wash the leaves and arrange on 4 serving plates.
2 Crush the garlic cloves and cut the chicken livers into small pieces.
3 Heat the oil in a frying pan, add the garlic and cook for a few seconds before adding the chicken livers. Fry quickly until the livers begin to brown and are just cooked.
4 Add the mustard and mix in.
5 Spoon the hot livers onto the salad, including any juices from the pan. Serve immediately.

Avocado and Cashew Nut Pâté

Serves 4

Butter beans could be used instead of the eggs, and other nuts could replace the cashew nuts.

1 ripe medium avocado	15ml/1 tbsp fresh parsley
15ml/1 tbsp lemon juice	4 black olives (optional)
55g/2 oz/½ cup cashew nuts	2 hardboiled eggs
1–2 spring onions (scallions)	black pepper

1 Mash the avocado and lemon juice with a fork.
2 Toast the cashew nuts, finely grind and allow to cool.
3 Finely chop the spring onion (scallion), parsley, olives and hard-boiled eggs by hand.
4 Mix all the ingredients together. Add a little water or soya milk if a softer pâté is required or if you wish to turn the pâté into a dip.
5 Serve with rice cakes, bread, vegetable crudités, salad etc.

Avocado Dip

Serves 4

Serve as a dip with vegetable crudités or as a pâté with rice cakes and a salad garnish. If desired, 15ml/1 tbsp of mayonnaise can be added.

1 clove garlic (optional)	pinch chilli powder
2 ripe avocados	3ml/½ tsp paprika
15ml/1 tbsp olive oil	black pepper
10ml/1 dsp lemon juice	

1 Press the garlic clove and place in a bowl with the other ingredients.
2 Mash with a fork to give a rough textured dip.

Carrot and Apricot Pâté

Serves 4–6

85g/3 oz/½ cup dried apricots	225g/8 oz/1⅓ cups grated carrot
90ml/3 fl oz/⅓ cup water	15ml/1 tbsp lemon juice
85g/3 oz/⅓ cup grated tofu	2ml/⅓ tsp cardamom
30g/1 oz/⅓ cup ground almonds	2ml/¼ tsp nutmeg
	black pepper

1 Cut the dried apricots into small pieces. Place in the water and simmer for 10 minutes or until soft.
2 Mix all the ingredients together by hand including any liquid remaining with the apricots.
3 Place in a small greased loaf tin, cover and bake for 45 minutes at 400°F/200°C/Gas Mark 6.
4 Cool a little, cut into slices and serve with a salad and rice cakes.

Carrot and Cashew Nut Pâté

Serves 4–6

Serve on rice cakes with a salad garnish or as a sandwich spread. For a variation, if allowed, add 40ml/2 tbsp cottage cheese and mix well.

255g/9 oz/1⅔ cups carrots, sliced	15ml/1 tbsp chopped chives *or* spring onion (scallion)
115g/4 oz/1 cup cashew nuts	black pepper
5ml/1 tsp chopped mint	approx. 15ml/1 tbsp orange
3ml/½ tsp grated orange rind	juice *or* soya milk

1 Slice and then cook the carrots in a little water until just soft. Sieve and cool.
2 Place the cashew nuts in a food processor and process until finely ground.
3 Add the carrots, mint, orange rind, onions or chives and pepper and process again. If necessary, add a little orange juice or milk to obtain a smooth pâté.

Butterbean, Tuna and Mint Pâté

Serves 4–6

1 tin 200g/7 oz/1⅓ cups tuna in water	15ml/1 tbsp olive oil
	15ml/1 tbsp lemon juice
225g/8 oz/1¼ cups cooked butterbeans	5ml/1 tsp fresh chopped mint
	black pepper

1 Drain the tuna, reserving the water, and place in the food processor with the remaining ingredients.
2 Process until smooth, adding a little of the tuna water if necessary to make a soft pâté. If you do not have a processor, mash the ingredients together in a bowl with a fork.

Humous and Crudités

Serves 4–6

Humous can be used as a pâté, a sandwich spread, a filling for baked potatoes or served with a selection of vegetable crudités as a dip. Crudités could include: sticks of carrot, celery, pepper and courgette (zucchini); broccoli and cauliflower florets and whole cherry tomatoes. I cheat if I am in a hurry and use tinned chickpeas.

225g/8 oz/1¼ cups cooked chickpeas	15ml/1 tbsp olive oil
	1 clove garlic (optional)
60ml/3 rounded tbsp tahini paste	2 spring onions (scallions)
	black pepper
30ml/2 tbsp lemon juice	a little water (if necessary)

1 Process all the ingredients until a soft, smooth pâté is obtained, using a little water if necessary.

Avocado and Tomato Starter

Serves 4

1 large avocado	80ml/4 tbsp sprouted seeds e.g.
1 large beef tomato	lentils, mung beans, aduki beans
salad leaves	60ml/4 tbsp French dressing
	(see Chapter 8, page 198)

1 Peel, halve and stone the avocado. Halve the tomato.
2 Lay both the tomato and the avocado halves cut side down and cut each half into 6 wedges.
3 On serving plates, arrange beds of salad leaves. On top, arrange alternate slices of avocado and tomato to form an upturned boat shape.
4 Sprinkle with sprouted seeds, and serve with French dressing.

Avocado and Mango Starter

Serves 4

Substitute mango for the tomato in the previous recipe. Arrange the avocado and mango in a fan shape. For special occasions, use the egg and prawn stuffing mixture from the Stuffed Lettuce Leaves recipe *(see page 71)* and pile at the point of each fan. Pour over the French dressing and, for those who can eat bread, use it to mop up the juices. Delicious!

Country Salad

This salad is delicious just as it is, but you can add cubes of creamy goat's cheese and serve with crusty bread, if your diet allows such luxuries.

455g/1 lb/3½ cups waxy new potatoes	4 spring onions (scallions) finely sliced
3 eggs, hardboiled	12 black olives (optional)
bunch asparagus *or* green beans	15ml/1 tbsp fresh parsley
1 large avocado	black pepper
½ red pepper, sliced	French dressing *(see Chapter 8,*
½ yellow pepper, sliced	*page 198)*
1 courgette (zucchini), thinly sliced	

1 Cook the potatoes whole and in their skins until tender. Cool. Peel off the skins if preferred. Cut into large chunks.
2 Shell and quarter the hardboiled eggs.
3 Steam the asparagus or beans for no longer than 5 minutes. Cool and slice into 3-cm/1-inch lengths.
4 Peel and stone the avocado and cut the flesh into chunks.
5 Gently layer the ingredients in a serving bowl so that they look mixed but have not been broken by the tossing.
6 Pour the French dressing over just before serving, or serve separately.

Savoury Fruit Salad

Serves 4–6

Other vegetables and fruit could be substituted in this recipe.

1 avocado	½ melon, cubed
15ml/1 tbsp lemon juice	½ cucumber, peeled and diced
30ml/2 tbsp olive oil	2 tomatoes, skinned and diced
black pepper	10ml/1 dsp chopped mint

1 Skin and stone the avocado and cut the flesh into cubes.
2 Mix together the lemon juice, olive oil and black pepper.
3 Place all the ingredients in a bowl and combine very gently.
4 If possible, chill for a few hours to allow the flavours to mingle.

Hors d'Oeuvres with Garlic Mayonnaise

Serves 4–6

mayonnaise (*see Chapter 8, page 200*)	Serve with a selection of the following: hardboiled eggs, tuna fish, sardines, baby sweetcorn, sugar snap peas, cooked broccoli, cherry tomatoes, whole radish, black olives, grilled peppers, cooked green beans
2 cloves garlic	
55g/2 oz/⅔ cup ground almonds	

1 Make the mayonnaise using half olive oil and half a lighter oil, such as sunflower.
2 Press the garlic cloves and add to the mayonnaise with the ground almonds. Mix well.
3 Serve to accompany a selection of the hors d'oeuvres.

Asparagus or Leeks with Walnut Mayonnaise

Serves 4

This is a delicious and unusual starter. Use a serrated knife for cutting the leeks; although not tough, they can be difficult to cut. The mayonnaise can be made by substituting 30ml/2 tbsp walnut oil for the other oils in the recipe.

1 bunch asparagus *or* 4 long thin young leeks	120ml/8 tbsp mayonnaise *(see Chapter 8, page 200)* 15g/½ oz/⅛ cup walnuts, finely chopped

1 If using the leeks, cut off and discard any green section. Halve each stem.
2 If using the asparagus, cut off the woody base of each stem.
3 Steam the leeks or asparagus for 5 minutes or until barely cooked. Cool quickly in cold water then drain.
4 Place the mayonnaise in a bowl and mix in most of the walnuts, reserving a few for garnishing.
5 Divide the leeks or asparagus between four plates and spoon the mayonnaise over the centre of each portion.
6 Garnish with the chopped walnuts.

SoupsSoupsSoupsSoupsSoupsSoups

Making soup is easy, as long as you have a good stock available. Instructions for making stock are given in the introduction *(see page 39)*. I always try to keep a supply of stock in the freezer, but do not be put off trying these recipes if you do not have ready-made stock as many are fine made with water. Those able to tolerate miso, shoyu/tamari sauce can use these to add extra flavour. However, avoid stock cubes in any form – I feel that the hydrolysed vegetable or meat protein which they contain is quite harmful.

A pan of soup is a useful standby. Served with a little rice, it makes an ideal mid-morning, afternoon or evening snack, and it can be used as a starter for lunch or evening meals.

Do not overcook soups. Beans and pulses obviously need cooking well but vegetables can be added at a later point and retain a better flavour and more vitamins if not overcooked. I rarely cook soups (except the beans) in a pressure cooker as it makes it too easy to over-cook them.

Try cutting vegetables into different shapes to produce different looking soups. For example, carrots can be finely diced, cut into match-stick pieces, sliced, grated, finely chopped in a food processor or left in rough chunks. Children will often eat soup more readily when it has been liquidized.

Pea Soup

Serves 4

Split peas could be used if a quicker version of this soup is required but I feel the whole peas give a nicer flavour. Soak the split peas for 2 hours and cook for approximately 45 minutes.

170g/6 oz/1 cup dried whole peas	3ml/½ tsp dried sage
1 litre/35 fl oz/4½ cups water *or* stock	2ml/¼ tsp dried thyme
	black pepper
1–2 sticks (stalks) celery	30ml/2 tbsp fresh parsley *or*
1 large onion	5ml/1 tsp dried

1 Soak the peas overnight in plenty of water.
2 Drain and rinse the peas. Cover with the stock or water, bring to the boil and simmer gently, covered with a lid, until soft and mushy. This will take approximately 1–1½ hours but only 10 minutes if using a pressure cooker. If not using a pressure cooker, you may need to add a little more water if the stock is evaporating.
3 Finely chop the celery and onion and add to the soup along with the dried sage, thyme, pepper and parsley. If using fresh parsley, add just before serving.
4 Bring to the boil and cook the soup for a further 15 minutes. Blend if a smoother soup is desired.

Light Lentil Soup

Serves 4

This is a soup I make when I am in a hurry as it is so quick and easy. It tastes fine even without stock.

115g/4 oz/½ cup red split lentils	5ml/1 tsp grated lemon rind
1 large onion	5ml/1tsp ground cumin
1 clove garlic	2ml/¼ tsp ground cloves
1 tin (400g/15 oz/2 cups) chopped tomatoes	1 bay leaf
850ml/1½ pints/3¾ cups stock *or* water	black pepper

1 Wash the lentils, finely chop the onion and press the garlic.
2 Place all the ingredients into a saucepan, bring to the boil, and simmer for 20–30 minutes.
3 Remove the bay leaf and serve.

Fennel, Celery and Leek Soup

Serves 4

Extra celery and leeks can be used if you do not have any fennel.

2 medium leeks	570ml/1 pint/2½ cups water
3–4 sticks (stalks) celery	425ml/15 fl oz/2 cups stock
1 large bulb fennel	285ml/10 fl oz/1⅓ cups soya *or*
10ml/1 dsp olive oil	almond milk
5ml/1 tsp fennel seeds	black pepper
5ml/1 tsp celery seeds	

1 Finely slice the leeks and celery and dice the fennel.
2 Heat the oil in a pan and add the vegetables plus the fennel and celery seeds. Sweat, stirring occasionally, until the vegetables are softened and beginning to brown.
3 Add the water, bring to the boil and simmer for 10 minutes.
4 Allow to cool a little then process until smooth. This stage can be omitted if you prefer a chunky soup or you do not have a food processor. Return the mixture to the pan.
5 Add the remaining ingredients and bring to the boil before serving.

Leekie Millet Broth

Serves 4

Oatflakes could be used instead of millet flakes if desired.

2 large leeks	3ml/½ tsp dried rosemary
2 large carrots	black pepper
570ml/1 pint/2½ cups stock	45g/1½ oz/½ cup millet flakes
570ml/1 pint/2½ cups water	140ml/5 fl oz/⅔ cup soya *or*
3ml/½ tsp dried thyme	almond milk

1 Slice the leeks and roughly chop the carrots.
2 Bring the stock and water to the boil and add the leeks, carrots, herbs and seasoning.
3 Bring to the boil again and simmer for 15 minutes.
4 Mix the millet flakes with the milk and stir into the soup. Bring to the boil, stirring until thickened, and simmer gently for 5 minutes before serving.

Carrot and Coriander Soup

If you do not have a food processor, or prefer your soup chunky, then grate the carrots and potato.

455g/1 lb/3¼ cups carrots	850ml/1½ pints/3¾ cups stock
1 large potato	black pepper
1 large onion	45ml/3 tbsp fresh *or* frozen
10ml/1 dsp olive oil	coriander

1 Slice the carrots and dice the potato and onion.
2 Sweat the onion and potato in the oil until they begin to soften and brown.
3 Add the carrots, the stock and the pepper. Bring to the boil and simmer for 10–15 minutes.
4 Process the soup, return to the pan, add the coriander, heat through and serve.

Carrot and Cardamom Soup

Serves 4

Substitute 55g/2 oz/¼ cup red split lentils for the potato in the previous recipe and add 3ml/½ tsp ground cardamom instead of or as well as the fresh coriander. Add the lentils along with the carrots and cook for 15 minutes.

Carrot and Tomato Soup

Serves 4

This is another soup I make if I'm in a hurry as it takes very little time to prepare and cook. If you do not have a food processor, finely grate the carrots and use ground almonds instead of the cashew nuts.

55g/2 oz/½ cup cashew nuts	3ml/½ tsp lemon rind
3 medium carrots	5ml/1 tsp mustard
570ml/1 pt/2½ cups stock *or* water	15ml/1 tbsp chopped fresh coriander
1 tin (400g/15 oz/2 cups) chopped tomatoes in juice	black pepper

1 Process the cashew nuts until finely ground. Add the carrots and process again until the carrots are finely chopped.
2 Place all the ingredients in a pan, bring to the boil and simmer for 10 minutes before serving.

Butterbean and Vegetable Soup

Serves 4

225g/8 oz/1 cup butter beans	2 leeks *or* onions
1 litre/35 fl oz/4½ cups stock *or* water	3ml/½ tsp dried thyme
2 large carrots	1 bayleaf
1 large parsnip	black pepper

1 Soak the butter beans overnight in lots of water.
2 Rinse the beans well and cook in the stock or water until soft, adding more water if the liquid is evaporating. To save time, use a pressure cooker if available and cook the beans for 10 minutes. The butter beans can be processed at this stage if a smoother soup is required.
3 Grate the carrots and parsnips and place in the pan with the beans.
4 Finely slice the leeks or onions and add to the pan along with the thyme, bayleaf and black pepper. Simmer for 15 minutes, remove the bayleaf and serve.

Quick Vegetable and Lentil Soup

Serves 4

1 large onion	2ml/¼ tsp dried marjoram
2 large carrots	2ml/¼ tsp dried oregano
1 large leek	2ml/¼ tsp dried rosemary
1 turnip	3ml/½ tsp paprika
3 sticks (stalks) celery	1ml/⅛ tsp cayenne pepper
1 clove garlic	1 bay leaf
115g/4 oz/½ cup red split lentils	black pepper
15ml/1 tbsp tomato purée (optional)	1½ litres/2½ pints/6 cups stock *or* water
3ml/½ tsp dried sage	

1 Cut all the vegetables into small pieces and press the garlic clove.
2 Place all the ingredients into a large pan, bring to the boil and simmer gently for 30 minutes. Remove the bay leaf.
3 Process if a smooth soup is required and serve.

Parsnip and Onion Soup

Serves 4

If you do not have a food processor, grate the parsnip and chop the onion very finely. For a creamier soup, add 140ml/5 fl oz/⅔ cup of soya milk.

2 medium parsnips	3ml/½ tsp garam masala
1 large onion	black pepper
10ml/1 dsp olive oil	1 litre/2 pts/5 cups stock
3ml/½ tsp curry powder	chopped walnuts to garnish

1 Dice the parsnips and onion and slowly sweat in the olive oil until they begin to brown, adding the spices and pepper for the last 2 minutes.
2 Add the stock and cook for 15 minutes.
3 Process the soup and serve with the walnuts floating on top.

Fish Soup

Serves 4

This is a lovely way to eat fish and is ideal for serving to those a little wary of eating fish or to children.

2 medium onions	juice of 1 orange
1 carrot	15ml/1 tbsp lemon juice
1 stick (stalk) celery	1 bay leaf
2 cloves garlic	black pepper
1 tin (400g/15 oz/2 cups) chopped tomatoes	455g/1 lb/2¾ cups cod *or* haddock
1 litre/35 fl oz/4½ cups fish stock *(see page 39)*	15ml/1 tbsp fresh parsley

1 Slice the onion, carrot and celery and press the garlic cloves.
2 Place all the ingredients except the fish and the parsley into a large pan. Bring to the boil and simmer for 10–15 minutes.
3 Cut or flake the fish into bite-sized pieces and add to the soup. Simmer for a further 5 minutes or until the fish is just cooked.
4 Serve sprinkled with parsley.

Cauliflower and Cashew Nut Soup

Serves 4

If you do not have a food processor, use ground almonds in place of the cashew nuts to thicken the soup.

1 onion	55g/2 oz/½ cup cashew nuts
1 leek	850ml/1½ pints/3¾ cups water
10ml/1 dsp olive oil	3ml/½ tsp curry powder
1 small cauliflower	2ml/¼ tsp thyme
1 large parsnip	3ml/½ tsp mustard
570ml/20 fl oz/2½ cups stock	black pepper

1 Chop the onion and leeks and sweat in the olive oil until they are soft.
2 Break the cauliflower into tiny florets, grate the parsnip and add to the pan along with the stock. Bring to the boil and then simmer for 10 minutes.
3 Process the cashew nuts until they are finely ground, then add half of the cauliflower mixture. Process again until smooth and creamy.
4 Return this mixture to the pan along with the remaining soup ingredients.
5 Bring to the boil and simmer for a further 5 minutes before serving.

Gazpacho

Serves 4

455g/1 lb/2¾ cups fresh
tomatoes
1 small green pepper
¼ small onion *or* 4 spring onions
(scallions)
½ large cucumber
20ml/2 dsp lemon juice

1 clove garlic (optional)
black pepper
10ml/1 dsp fresh chopped
parsley
10ml/1 dsp fresh chopped mint
extra parsley to garnish

1 Skin the tomatoes by placing in boiling water for approximately 1 minute.
2 Roughly cut the vegetables, then process all the ingredients until a smooth mixture is obtained.
3 Serve chilled, garnished with parsley.

Leek, Sweetcorn and Almond Soup

Serves 4

Use peas if you cannot tolerate corn. If you do not have a food processor, use ground almonds to thicken the soup.

1 large onion	570ml/1 pint/2½ cups stock
680g/1½ lb/6 cups leeks	170g/6 oz/1 cup sweetcorn
3 sticks (stalks) celery	kernels
10ml/1 dsp olive oil	3ml/½ tsp mustard (optional)
85g/3 oz/½ cup whole almonds	10ml/1 dsp fresh parsley
850ml/1½ pints/3¾ cups water	black pepper

1 Chop the onions, leeks and celery then sweat in the oil until the vegetables are soft and beginning to brown.
2 Process the almonds until finely ground, then add half the vegetable mixture and approximately 285ml/½ pt/1⅓ cups of water. Process again until smooth and creamy.
3 Return this mixture to the pan along with the remaining ingredients.
4 Bring the soup to the boil and simmer for 10 minutes before serving.

Majorcan Soup

This is my version of a soup I had while on holiday in Majorca. It looked disappointing when it arrived but it turned out to be delicious, despite its simple ingredients. It is a thick stew-type of soup but could be served watered down with more stock if desired.

2 onions
225g/½ lb/4 cups white cabbage
15ml/1 tbsp olive oil
170g/6 oz/1½ cups mangetout
or green beans

black pepper
425ml/15 fl oz/2 cups good
quality stock

1 Roughly chop the onions and cabbage and sweat them in the olive oil until they begin to soften and brown.
2 Add the beans or mangetout, the pepper and the stock, bring to the boil and simmer for 10 minutes before serving.

Chicken and Seaweed Broth

Serves 4

I make this soup whenever I have the remains of a chicken carcass, but it can be made without the chicken by substituting vegetable stock.

1 chicken carcass	10ml/1 dsp olive oil
1¾ litres/3 pints/7½ cups water	2 strips wakame seaweed
2 onions	10ml/1 dsp tomato purée
2 carrots	(optional)
3 sticks (stalks) celery	black pepper

1 Cover the carcass with the water, bring to the boil and simmer for 45 minutes.
2 Remove any meat from the carcass and keep to one side. Discard the carcass.
3 Sieve the stock and preferably leave to stand overnight in the fridge to allow any fat to come to the surface.
4 Remove any fat from the stock by laying kitchen paper on the surface and allowing it to soak up the fat.
5 Chop the onions, carrots and celery and sweat in the oil until they begin to soften and brown.
6 Cut the wakame seaweed into small pieces using kitchen scissors. Soak the seaweed in a little water to soften, if necessary. Add to the pan along with the tomato purée and the black pepper.
7 Simmer for 15 minutes before serving.

SaladsSaladsSaladsSaladsSaladsSal

When you mention a salad to most people it conjures up images of lettuce, tomato and cucumber and pangs of hunger for the rest of the afternoon or evening.

Salads need not be so. There is such a wide variety of vegetables, fruit and nuts which can be used that they need never be boring. Neither do they need to be lacking in substance. I never serve the typical lettuce, tomato and cucumber salad except as a side dish to accompany a substantial meal. Serve instead a selection of salads as a main course so that people can help themselves and pile their plates high. Any leftovers can be used for lunch the next day. In winter, serve a warm soup as a starter and a baked potato or hot rice dish with the salads.

Salads are easy to make because the quantity of ingredients is not that important. If you do not have all the ingredients for the following recipes, substitute your favourite ingredients or whatever you have available. You can go on inventing new salads for ever.

Salads make ideal starters. If you want a two-course meal or feel you eat insufficient raw food then try serving some of the following salads as starters.

The following recipes all serve at least four adults and in many cases there will be some left over for lunch the next day.

A VARIETY OF SALADS

A delicious meal can be produced by making lots of different salads out of whatever ingredients you have available. Do not worry about the quantities and use fresh fruit, dried fruit, nuts and seeds as well as vegetables and herbs. Dressings could include mayonnaise *(see page 200)*, soya yogurt and French dressing *(see page 198),* where appropriate. Try to group ingredients so that colours, flavours and textures complement each other.

Following are suggestions and approximate quantities. The ingredients just need mixing. Omit the French dressing if desired.

Tuna and Bean Salad

1 tin (200g/7 oz/1⅓ cups) tuna
115g/4 oz/⅔ cup red kidney
beans
diced flesh of 1 small orange

55g/2 oz/½ cup toasted cashew
nuts
15ml/1 tbsp French dressing
(optional)

Avocado and Grapefruit Salad

diced flesh of 1 red grapefruit
diced flesh of 1 ripe avocado
5ml/1 tsp grated ginger

225g/8 oz/4 cups spinach
leaves, chopped

Courgette (Zucchini) and Cauliflower Salad

2 courgettes (zucchini), sliced
½ small cauliflower, broken into
small florets

5ml/1 tsp caraway seeds,
mayonnaise or French dressing

Beansprout and Sweetcorn Salad

55g/2 oz/⅔ cup beansprouts
115g/4 oz/½ cup sweetcorn
kernels

½ diced cucumber
2 tomatoes, skinned and diced

Root Vegetable and Raisin Salad

1 grated turnip, celeriac *or* kohlrabi	30ml/2 tbsp raisins
1 large grated carrot	30ml/2 tbsp French dressing *or* orange juice

Apple, Celery and Beetroot Salad

1 large cooked beetroot, cubed	15ml/1 tbsp chopped walnuts
1 stick (stalk) celery, diced	15ml/1 tbsp French dressing
1 eating apple, sliced (leave the skin on)	

Bean and Pepper Salad

225g/8 oz/1¼ cups mixed beans	½ red pepper, diced
2 chopped spring onions (scallions)	15ml/1 tbsp fresh herbs
	15ml/1 tbsp French dressing

Bean and Sweetcorn Salad

225g/8 oz/1¼ cups red kidney beans	225g/8 oz/1¼ cups sweetcorn kernels
170g/6 oz/2 cups cooked green beans (cut into 2.5-cm/1-inch lengths)	

Carrot and Beetroot Salad

225g/8 oz/1⅓ cups grated raw carrot

225g/8 oz/1⅓ cups grated raw beetroot

2 sticks (stalks) celery, diced

30ml/2 tbsp sultanas (optional)

30ml/2 tbsp French dressing

Avocado, Smoked Tofu and Pineapple Salad

diced flesh of 1 large avocado

1 cup chopped pineapple

170g/6 oz/1 cup diced smoked tofu

Beetroot and Pineapple Salad

5 medium beetroot, diced

30ml/2 tbsp chopped walnuts

8 pitted prunes, chopped (optional)

1 cup chopped pineapple

10ml/1 dsp lemon juice

Rice, Sweetcorn and Bean Salad

115g/4 oz/⅔ cup cooked brown rice

55g/2 oz/⅓ cup sweetcorn *or* peas

55g/2 oz/⅓ cup red kidney beans

15ml/1 tbsp fresh herbs (mint, parsley, chives etc.)

15ml/1 tbsp French dressing

Rice and Carrot Salad

115g/4 oz/⅔ cup cooked brown rice
1 grated carrot
1 stick (stalk) celery, diced
3 radishes, sliced

2 spring onions (scallions), sliced
30ml/2 tbsp toasted sunflower seeds
15ml/1 tbsp fresh herbs
15ml/1 tbsp French dressing

Hazelnut and Rice Salad

170g/6 oz/1 cup cooked brown rice
3ml/½ tsp ground cinnamon
30ml/2 tbsp toasted sesame seeds
30ml/2 tbsp raisins (optional)

30ml/2 tbsp toasted, chopped hazelnuts
6 chopped dried apricots (optional)
30ml/2 tbsp French dressing
5ml/1 tsp grated ginger

Leaf Greens, Arame and Satsuma Salad

chopped greens (lettuce, spinach, Chinese leaves, watercress)
2 satsumas, segmented

30g/1 oz/½ cup arame seaweed soaked in water until soft
French dressing

Broccoli and Red Bean Salad

340g/12 oz/4 cups broccoli florets (slightly cooked)
115g/4 oz/⅔ cup red kidney beans

2 sticks (stalks) celery, sliced
2 spring onions (scallions), sliced
French dressing

Pineapple and Olive Salad

salad greens (Chinese leaves, spinach, cress)
12 black olives
½ cup pineapple pieces

2 tomatoes, cut into segments
5-cm/2-inch piece cucumber, cubed

Avocado, Sweetcorn and Olive Salad

1 avocado, diced
12 black olives, halved

115g/4 oz/½ cup sweetcorn *or* peas
15ml/1 tbsp French dressing

The following salads also make excellent accompaniments to curries.

Cucumber, Mint and Yogurt Salad

½ cucumber, peeled and diced
15ml/1 tbsp chopped mint

2.5-cm/1-inch piece ginger, grated
140ml/5 fl oz/⅔ cup soya yogurt

Tomato and Coriander Salad

5 large tomatoes, skinned and sliced
2 spring onions (scallions), finely sliced

15ml/1 tbsp chopped fresh coriander
French dressing

Apple, Carrot and Ginger Salad

1 grated apple	10ml/1 dsp grated ginger
1 large grated carrot	15ml/1 tbsp French dressing

All in One Salad

One of my favourite meals is a bowl of salad which contains anything I have available. Serve this on its own, with baked potatoes, boiled new potatoes or with a savoury rice salad.

In a large bowl put *any* of the following ingredients in *any* quantities until you have sufficient salad. Mix gently and serve, dressed if you like with French dressing:

- shredded lettuce, spinach, Chinese leaves, white cabbage *or* red cabbage
- grated carrot, parsnip, celeriac *or* kohlrabi
- diced cucumber, avocado, pepper, tomato, fennel, peach *or* apple
- sliced celery, radish, spring onion (scallion) *or* courgette (zucchini)
- florets of cauliflower and broccoli
- sweetcorn kernels, fresh peas, broad beans, olives *or* grapes
- cooked beans e.g. chickpeas *or* red kidney beans
- chopped, flaked *or* toasted nuts and seeds
- fresh herbs e.g. mint, chives, parsley
- watercress, mustard cress, sprouted seeds.

Coleslaw

An alternative coleslaw can be made by adding 80ml/4 rounded tbsp mayonnaise instead of the dressing *(see page 200).*

225g/8 oz/4 cups white cabbage	DRESSING
½ bulb fennel *or* 2 sticks (stalks) celery	45ml/3 tbsp olive oil
1 small eating apple	1 spring onion (scallion), finely sliced
1 large carrot	3ml/½ tsp mustard
20ml/1 tbsp sultanas	15ml/1 tbsp lemon juice
40ml/2 tbsp chopped walnuts	3ml/½ tsp grated ginger

1 Shred the cabbage and fennel finely. Chop the celery and the unpeeled apple. Grate the carrot.
2 Shake the dressing ingredients together in a screw-topped jar.
3 Mix all the coleslaw ingredients and the dressing together in a bowl.

Curried Apple Coleslaw

If preferred, a French dressing could be used instead of the mayonnaise and yogurt.

225g/8 oz/4 cups white cabbage	DRESSING
8 radishes	60ml/3 rounded tbsp mayonnaise *(see page 200)*
2 large sticks (stalks) celery	60ml/3 rounded tbsp soya
2 spring onions (scallions)	yogurt *or* extra mayonnaise
1 red eating apple	10ml/1 dsp lemon juice
10ml/2 tsp caraway seeds	3 ml/½ tsp curry powder

1 Shred the cabbage. Slice the radishes, the celery, the spring onions (scallions) and the unpeeled apple.
2 Mix the dressing ingredients together.
3 Combine all the ingredients in a large bowl.

Minted Avocado and Chickpea Salad

This salad makes a lovely starter served on a bed of crisp lettuce.

115g/4 oz/½ cup chickpeas	15ml/1 tbsp lemon juice
1 large banana	5ml/1 tsp fresh mint
1 medium ripe avocado	1 clove garlic, optional
60ml/3 rounded tbsp mayonnaise *(see page 200)*	paprika to garnish

1 Cook the chickpeas until tender and allow to cool.
2 Slice the banana and dice the avocado flesh into a bowl. Toss gently in the lemon juice.
3 Stir in the remaining ingredients and garnish with paprika.

Chicken, Egg, Almond and Potato Salad

Avocado can be used if you cannot tolerate eggs, and cooked butter beans can be substituted for the chicken.

225g/8 oz/2 cups new potatoes
115g/4 oz/1 cup cooked chicken
2 hardboiled eggs

80ml/4 rounded tbsp mayonnaise *(see page 200)*
55g/2 oz/½ cup toasted flaked almonds

1 Cook the potatoes in their skins and, when cool, skin and dice.
2 Roughly chop the chicken and hardboiled eggs.
3 Mix all the ingredients together.

Tuna and Celery Salad

2 sticks (stalks) celery
225g/8 oz/1½ cups cooked rice
1 tin (200g/7 oz/1⅓ cups) tuna in water

mayonnaise *(see page 200),* soya yogurt *or* French dressing *(see page 198)*

1 Finely dice the celery and combine with the rice and drained tuna.
2 Use sufficient French dressing, mayonnaise or yogurt to bind the ingredients. I like to use a mixture of yogurt and mayonnaise.

Jellied Beetroot Salad

Gelozone is the vegetarian alternative to gelatine.

285ml/½ pint/1⅓ cups orange juice
3g/1 level tsp Gelozone

340g/12 oz/2 cups cooked beetroot

1 Pour the fruit juice into a pan and sprinkle the Gelozone on top. Stir until dissolved. Bring the mixture to the boil, stirring all the time.
2 Cube the beetroot and add to the pan. Mix.
3 Pour into a serving dish and refrigerate until set and cold.

Jellied Carrot Salad

Follow the previous recipe but add 225g/8 oz/1⅓ cups finely grated raw carrot instead of the beetroot. Try other flavoured fruit juices.

Millet Tabouli

Tabouli is traditionally made with couscous which is made from wheat. Use this, if you are allowed, as it is delicious. Just add the uncooked couscous to the salad instead of the millet. It will soften by soaking up the juices. Allow to stand for 2 hours before serving.

85g/3 oz/½ cup whole millet	10ml/1 dsp chopped chives *or*
4 large tomatoes	spring onions (scallions)
¼ red pepper	30ml/2 tbsp fresh chopped mint
¼ cucumber	(essential)
1 stick (stalk) celery	30ml/2 tbsp French dressing
15ml/1 tbsp chopped parsley	*(see page 198)*

1 Cook the millet in 425ml/¾ pint/2 cups of boiling water for approximately 18 minutes. Sieve the millet and allow to cool.
2 Skin and finely chop the tomatoes. Finely dice the pepper, cucumber and celery.
3 Mix the millet, salad vegetables, herbs and French dressing together and leave to stand for a few hours to allow the flavours to mingle.

Mediterranean Lentil Salad

170g/6 oz/1 cup whole lentils | 1 small carrot
1 orange | ¼ red pepper
1 clove garlic | ¼ green pepper
30ml/2 tbsp olive oil | 2 spring onions (scallions)
15ml/1 tbsp lemon juice | 5ml/1 tsp fresh parsley, chives
3ml/½ tsp lemon rind | and mint
3ml/½ tsp orange rind | 40ml/2 tbsp currants, optional

1 Cook the lentils for approximately 15–20 minutes in lots of water until soft but not mushy. Drain.
2 Dice the orange flesh and press the garlic clove.
3 Add to the lentils along with the oil, lemon juice and the orange and lemon rind whilst the lentils are still warm. Allow to cool.
4 Grate the carrot, dice the peppers, slice the spring onions (scallions) and finely chop the herbs.
5 When cool, combine all the salad ingredients and, if possible, stand for 1 hour before serving to allow the flavours to mix.

Rice Pilaf Ring

Serve as it is or fill the centre with Tropical Curried Chicken Salad *(page 117)* or Minted Avocado and Chickpea Salad *(page 110)*. The French dressing can be omitted – the pilaf should still stick together provided the rice has been cooked sufficiently.

1 large onion	570ml/1 pint/2½ cups water
15ml/1 tbsp olive oil	3ml/½ tsp cinnamon
225g/8 oz/1 cup brown rice	1 bay leaf
45g/1½ oz/¼ cup dried apricots	black pepper
55g/2 oz/½ cup walnuts	30ml/2 tbsp French dressing
45g/1½ oz/¼ cup raisins	*(see page 198)*

1 Dice the onion and sweat in the oil for approximately 10 minutes.
2 Soak the rice in cold water for 15 minutes. Rinse and drain.
3 Finely chop the apricots and walnuts and add to the pan with the rice, the raisins, the water and the herbs and spices.
4 Bring to the boil, cover and simmer for approximately 40 minutes until the rice is cooked and all the water has been absorbed. If necessary, add a little more water during cooking.
5 Remove the bay leaf and stir in the French dressing while still warm. Press into a ring mould and leave to cool.

Red Cabbage Salad

This dish can be served hot as a vegetable or allowed to cool and served as a salad. It can be cooked on the top of the stove, but be careful as it will quickly dry out and burn.

455g/1 lb/8 cups red cabbage	juice of 1 orange
1 onion	10ml/1 dsp lemon juice
1 large baking apple	3ml/½ tsp orange rind
40ml/2 tbsp raisins, optional	3ml/½ tsp lemon rind
60ml/2 fl oz/¼ cup water	

1 Chop the red cabbage, slice the onion and grate the apple.
2 Mix all the ingredients together in a casserole dish. Cover and cook in the oven at 400°F/200°C/Gas Mark 6 for approximately 1 hour, stirring once during cooking.

Curried Egg and Rice Salad

Avocado can be substituted for the hardboiled eggs.

170g/6 oz/¾ cup brown rice	4 hardboiled eggs
1 medium onion	60ml/3 rounded tbsp
5 ml/1 tsp curry powder	mayonnaise (see page 200)
5ml/1 tsp paprika	60ml/3 tbsp soya yogurt or
10ml/1 dsp tomato purée	extra mayonnaise

1 Cook the rice and allow to cool.
2 Finely dice the onion and cook in 30ml/2 tbsp water for 5 minutes.
3 Stir the curry powder, paprika and tomato purée into the onions and allow to cool.
4 Coarsely chop the hardboiled eggs, then stir all the ingredients gently together.

Tropical Curried Chicken Salad

This makes a delicious filling for the Rice Pilaf Ring *(page 115)* or it can be served as one of a selection of salads or as a starter on a bed of lettuce garnished with toasted coconut. Vegetarians could substitute butter beans for the chicken.

2 bananas	DRESSING
15ml/1 tbsp lemon juice	2 spring onions
340g/12 oz/2½ cups cooked chicken	¼ eating apple
55g/2 oz/¼ cup dried apricots	3ml/½ tsp curry powder
55g/2 oz/⅓ cup toasted cashews	3ml/½ tsp lemon juice
30g/1 oz/⅙ cup sultanas, optional	80ml/4 rounded tbsp mayonnaise *(see page 200)*

1 To make the dressing, slice the spring onions and finely grate the apple before combining the dressing ingredients.
2 Slice the bananas and toss in the lemon juice to prevent browning.
3 Cut the chicken into bite-sized chunks and dice the apricots into small pieces.
4 Place all the ingredients together and gently mix with the dressing.

MainlyVegetarianMainlyVegetaria

Vegetable Chilli with Walnuts and Quinoa

Serves 4

If you do not have a food processor, use ground almonds instead of ground walnuts. Millet could be used instead of the quinoa, and other favourite vegetables substituted.

115g/4 oz/⅔ cup quinoa	225g/8 oz/1⅓ cups cooked red
1 onion	kidney beans
1 carrot	570ml/1 pt/2½ cups carrot *or*
2 sticks (stalks) celery	tomato juice
15ml/1 tbsp olive oil	juice and rind of 1 orange
2 courgettes (zucchini)	3ml/½ tsp nutmeg
½ red pepper	10ml/1 dsp paprika
115g/4 oz/1 cup walnut halves	black pepper

1 Cook the quinoa in 425ml/¾ pint/2 cups boiling water for 15 minutes.
2 Dice the onion, carrot and celery, and sweat in the oil until they begin to soften and brown.
3 Finely dice the courgettes (zucchini) and the red pepper. Add to the pan along with the other vegetables, and continue to sweat until they are beginning to soften.
4 Process two-thirds of the walnuts until they are finely ground, and add these to the vegetables along with the remaining walnuts broken into smaller pieces and the quinoa mixture.
5 Add the remaining ingredients, mix well and spoon into a large, shallow gratin dish. Bake uncovered in the centre of the oven at 400°F/200°C/Gas Mark 6 for 30 minutes.

Lentil Bolognese

Serves 4

Serve with rice or pasta, as a filling for baked potatoes, as a stuffing for vegetables, taco shells or in a lasagne. I always make up double the quantity of this recipe as it freezes well and is a super standby. If tomatoes are not tolerated, use carrot juice.

115g/4 oz/⅔ cup brown lentils	570ml/1 pt/2½ cups creamed
1 onion	tomatoes *or* tomato juice
½ green pepper	5ml/1 tsp dried oregano
1 stick (stalk) celery	5ml/1 tsp dried basil
1 carrot	1 bay leaf
2 cloves garlic	black pepper
285ml/½ pt/1⅓ cups water	

1 Wash the lentils well.
2 Finely chop the onion, green pepper and celery. Dice the carrot and press the garlic cloves.
3 Place all the ingredients into a pan, bring to the boil and simmer, covered, for 30 minutes or until the lentils are soft but not mushy.

Lentil Moussaka

Serves 4

1 portion Lentil Bolognese *(see page 121)*	1 aubergine (eggplant)
3 courgettes (zucchini)	680g/1½ lb/5 cups potatoes
	10ml/1 dsp olive oil

1 Place half the lentil mix into a large, shallow ovenproof dish.
2 Cut the courgettes (zucchini) and aubergine (eggplant) into 1½-cm/½-inch slices and place in layers on top of the lentils. Cover with the remaining lentil mix.
3 Peel the potatoes and cut into ¼-cm/⅛-inch slices, using a food processor if available. Layer these on top of the lentils and vegetables.
4 Brush the top with olive oil and bake at 400°F/200°C/Gas Mark 6 for 1¼ hours until the potatoes are cooked and crisp.

Vegetarian Shepherds Pie

Serves 4

An alternative topping could be made by mixing cooked millet and mashed parsnips in roughly equal quantities.

| 680g/1½ lb/5 cups potatoes | *page 121)* |
| 1 portion Lentil Bolognese *(see* | 10ml/1 dsp olive oil |

1 Cook the potatoes until soft and mash with a small amount of the cooking liquid or a little soya milk, until light and fluffy.
2 Place the Lentil Bolognese into a shallow ovenproof dish.
3 Spread the potatoes on top, level the surface and brush with olive oil.
4 Bake for 45 minutes at 400°F/200°C/Gas Mark 6. Place under the grill for a few minutes if the surface has not browned sufficiently.

Fruit & Nut Slices (p213) *with* **Strawberry Fruit Fool (p247)** *and* **Popcorn (p226)**

**Vegetable Risotto
(p134)** *with* **Avocado &
Tomato Starter (p78)**

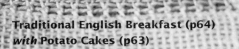
Traditional English Breakfast (p64)
with Potato Cakes (p63)

Sweet Soufflé Omelette (p252) filled with fresh summer fruits and served with Banana & Mango Ice Cream (p251)

**Lentil Bolognese (p121)
served in Taco Shells
with Leaf Greens, Arame
& Satsuma Salad (p106)**

Carrot & Coriander Soup (p89) *with*
Onion & Herb Focaccia Bread (p222)

**Chicken with Barbecue
Sauce (p169) and wild rice
with Asparagus & Walnut
Mayonnaise (p81)**

Peppered Cod (p184) served
with Carrot & Coconut Rice
(p156) *and* Broccoli & Red
Bean Salad (p106)

Carrot and Courgette (Zucchini) Bake

Serves 4

Serve with baked potatoes and a selection of salads.

1 onion, diced	30g/1 oz/⅙ cup rice flour
10ml/1 dsp olive oil	115ml/4 fl oz/½ cup soya *or*
2 courgettes (zucchini), grated	almond milk
2 carrots, grated	3ml/½ tsp baking powder
2 eggs	3ml/½ tsp dried rosemary
55g/2 oz/⅓ cup maize meal *or*	3ml/½ tsp dried thyme
polenta flour	black pepper

1 Sweat the onion in the oil until it begins to soften and brown.
2 Mix in a bowl the onion, courgettes (zucchini) and carrots.
3 Beat the eggs with the maize meal, rice flour, milk, baking powder, herbs and black pepper. Combine the two mixtures.
4 Pour into a greased gratin dish and bake uncovered at 400°F/ 200°C/Gas Mark 6 for 45 minutes to 1 hour or until brown and set.

Millet and Walnut Bake

Serves 4

Serve hot with salads, vegetables or baked potatoes.

Other vegetables can be substituted for a variation.

The original recipe for this dish uses couscous instead of millet. If you are allowed wheat, try it, as it really does make a delicious bake. Just add 85g/3 oz/½ cup of couscous along with the remaining ingredients, and add a total of 850ml/1½ pints/3¾ cups of liquid, including the vegetable juice. The couscous will soak up the liquid as it cooks. A little grated cheese on top of this dish will make even the most ardent meat-eaters start thinking vegetarian.

570ml/1 pt/2½ cups tomato, carrot *or* vegetable juice	2 medium courgettes (zucchini)
570ml/1 pt/2½ cups water	115g/4 oz/1 cup walnuts
115g/4 oz/⅔ cup millet grain	15ml/1 tbsp olive oil
1 onion	3 ml/½ tsp dried thyme
1 large stick (stalk) celery	3ml/½ tsp dried rosemary
1 carrot	black pepper

1 Mix the vegetable juice and the water and cook the millet for 20 minutes in 570ml/1 pint/2½ cups of this liquid.
2 Finely chop the onion and celery, finely dice the carrot and courgettes (zucchini). Process the walnuts in a food processor until they are roughly ground.
3 Sweat the onion, carrot and celery in the oil until they start to soften and brown. Add the courgettes (zucchini) and sweat for a few more minutes.
4 Add the millet mixture, the remaining liquid, the nuts, herbs and pepper.
5 Mix well and place in a large, shallow, ovenproof dish.
6 Bake uncovered in the centre of the oven for 30 minutes at 400°F/200°C/Gas Mark 6.

Cauliflower and Courgette Bake

Serves 4

Serve hot with potatoes or rice and salads or vegetables.

680g/1½ lb/6 cups cauliflower, divided into florets	140ml/5 fl oz/⅔ cup soya *or* almond milk
2 courgettes (zucchini)	3 eggs, separated
45ml/3 tbsp rice flour	10ml/1 dsp olive oil
5ml/1 tsp mustard	

1 Cook the cauliflower for approximately 5 minutes in boiling water until just tender.
2 Cut the courgettes (zucchini) into 1-cm/¼-inch slices.
3 Mix the flour and mustard with the milk in a pan and bring gently to the boil, stirring all the time. Simmer for 1 minute. The sauce will be very thick.
4 Blend the cauliflower, egg yolks and white sauce in a food processor until smooth.
5 Whisk the egg whites until stiff and fold into the cauliflower mixture with a large metal spoon.
6 Spoon half the mixture into a greased gratin dish. Arrange half the courgettes (zucchini) on top, then cover with the remaining cauliflower mixture. Top with the remaining courgette (zucchini) and brush with olive oil.
7 Bake at 400°F/200°C/Gas Mark 6 for approximately 30 minutes or until golden brown and set.

Savoury Pancakes

Serves 4

Stuffed pancakes take a little time to prepare but are worth the effort for special meals. Even confirmed meat-eaters will love them. To save time, pancakes can be made in bulk and frozen.

1 egg	60ml/2 fl oz/¼ cup water
115g/4 oz/⅔ cup rice flour	170ml/6 fl oz/¾ cup soya milk
5ml/1 level tsp baking powder	10ml/1 dsp olive oil

1 Blend all the ingredients except the oil in the food processor. If mixing by hand, beat the egg then add the remaining ingredients except the oil and beat well.
2 Oil a griddle or frying pan and cook 4 large or 8 small pancakes. Turn as soon as the pancakes are puffed and full of bubbles.

Ratatouille-Stuffed Pancakes

Fill the pancakes with Ratatouille *(see Chapter 8, page 203)* and place in one large or four small gratin dishes. Cover with White Sauce *(see Chapter 8, page 201)* and sprinkle the surface with chopped nuts or, if allowed, a mixture of breadcrumbs and grated cheese. Place in a hot oven or under the grill to warm through and brown.

Lentil Bolognese Pancakes

Follow the above recipe but use the Lentil Bolognese ingredients to stuff the pancakes *(see page 121)*.

Carrot, Butterbean and Walnut Pancakes

Cook 565g (1¼ lbs) carrots until tender, then mash with ½ tsp orange rind, some black pepper and sufficient cooking liquid to make a soft purée. Add 170g (6oz/¾ cup) cooked butterbeans and 55g (2oz/⅔ cup) walnuts. Fill the pancakes with this mixture, as above, then coat with a white sauce *(see page 201).*

Celeriac and Sweetcorn Pancakes

Cook 565g (1¼ lbs) celeriac until tender and mash with ¼ tsp ground nutmeg, some black pepper and sufficient soya milk to make a soft purée. Add 225g (8oz/1¼ cups) cooked sweetcorn. Fill the pancakes with this mixture, as above, and coat with white sauce *(see page 201).*

Black Eyed Bean and Vegetable Terrine

Serves 4

Serve hot or cold with a selection of vegetables or salads. Substitute cooked millet or quinoa for the rice if desired.

170g/6 oz/1 cup black eyed beans	10ml/1 dsp fresh parsley
1 large onion	10ml/1 dsp fresh coriander
2 sticks (stalks) celery	115g/4 oz/⅔ cup cooked rice
1 courgette (zucchini)	3ml/½ tsp grated lemon rind
1 medium carrot	5ml/1 tsp grated ginger
1 clove garlic	3ml/½ tsp dried basil
10ml/1 dsp olive oil	2ml/¼ tsp dried thyme
	black pepper

1 Soak the black eyed beans overnight. Rinse and then cook in lots of water until quite soft. Sieve to remove the cooking liquid.
2 Finely dice the onion, celery and courgette (zucchini), grate the carrot and press the garlic clove. Sweat the onion, celery and garlic in the oil until they begin to soften and brown. Add the courgette (zucchini) and carrot and continue cooking until they too begin to soften.
3 Finely chop the parsley and coriander and place in a bowl along with the rest of the ingredients. Mix together but do not be gentle as the beans should partially break up, making the mixture quite soft.
4 Place in a greased loaf tin and bake in the centre of the oven at 400°F/200°C/Gas Mark 6 for approximately 45 minutes or until the loaf is beginning to brown around the edges.

Nutty Vegetable Loaf

Serves 4

Serve hot with vegetables, salads, rice or potatoes and with a sauce from Chapter 8, such as Fresh Tomato *(see page 204)*, Onion *(see page 201)* or Vegetable Purée *(see page 205)*. Alternatively, serve cold with a selection of salads. You can replace the tomato purée with 5ml/1 tsp miso, and the vegetables can also be varied.

1 onion	10ml/1 dsp tomato purée
½ red pepper	2ml/¼ tsp dried thyme
10ml/1 dsp olive oil	2ml/¼ tsp dried rosemary
1 medium carrot, grated	2ml/¼ tsp nutmeg
½ medium baking apple, grated	1ml/⅛ tsp cayenne pepper
115g/4 oz/⅔ cup cooked brown rice, buckwheat *or* millet	5ml/1 tsp mustard, optional
55g/2 oz/½ cup nuts, finely ground, e.g. hazelnuts, walnuts	black pepper

1 Finely dice the onion and red pepper, and sweat in the oil until they soften and begin to brown.
2 Add the grated carrot and apple and sweat for another few minutes until they too begin to soften.
3 Combine all the ingredients and mix well.
4 Place the mixture in a greased loaf tin and bake covered for approximately 40 minutes in the centre of the oven at 400°F/200°C/Gas Mark 6.

Squirrel's Delight

Serves 4

Serve hot with vegetables, salads, rice or potatoes and with a sauce from Chapter 8, such as Fresh Tomato *(see page 204)*, Onion *(see page 201)* or Vegetable Purée *(see page 205)*.

1 onion	115g/4 oz/⅔ cup cooked millet, rice, quinoa *or* buckwheat
1 stick (stalk) celery	
55g/2 oz/½ cup mushrooms (optional)	15ml/1 tbsp fresh chopped coriander
1 clove garlic	30ml/2 tbsp fresh chopped parsley
10ml/1 dsp olive oil	
55g/2 oz/½ cup chopped almonds	10ml/1 dsp lemon juice
	3ml/½ tsp grated lemon rind
85g/3 oz/¾ cup chopped cashews	3ml/½ level tsp cinnamon
	5ml/1 level tsp ground coriander
30g/1 oz/⅓ cup ground almonds	2ml/¼ tsp fennel seeds
2 eggs *or* an egg replacer	2 pinches ground cloves
60ml/3 tbsp sweetcorn *or* peas	black pepper

1 Finely dice the onion, celery and mushrooms and press the garlic clove.
2 Sweat the onion, garlic and celery in the oil until they soften and begin to brown. Add the mushrooms and sweat for 2 minutes.
3 Mix all the ingredients together.
4 Place in a greased loaf tin and cover with foil.
5 Bake at 400°F/200°C/Gas Mark 6 for approximately 45 minutes. For a more moist loaf steam over a pan of water for 45 minutes or pressure cook for 15 minutes.

Nut Roast

Serves 4

This loaf remains moist because of the way it is cooked. It can be served hot and is delicious with the Orange and Ginger Sauce from the Vegetable and Fruit Kebab recipe *(see page 132)*. However, it can also be served cold with salads or as a pâté.

The original recipe contained 55g/2 oz/1 cup of breadcrumbs instead of the rice, so try this as a variation if your diet allows bread. If permitted, use 3ml/½ tsp miso to make a tasty stock.

1 small onion	2ml/¼ tsp dried thyme
2 large mushrooms *or* 1 stick (stalk) celery	30g/1 oz/¼ cup almonds
	55g/2 oz/½ cup hazelnuts
1 large tomato	30g/1 oz/¼ cup cashews
10ml/1 dsp olive oil	115g/4 oz/⅔ cup cooked rice,
10ml/1 level dsp rice flour	millet *or* quinoa
90ml/3 fl oz/⅓ cup water *or* stock	1 egg (optional)
2ml/¼ tsp dried rosemary	black pepper

1 Finely dice the onion, mushrooms (or celery), and skin and dice the tomato.
2 Sweat the onion in the oil until soft. Add the mushrooms or celery and cook for 2–3 minutes. Stir in the tomato, cover and simmer for 3 minutes.
3 Sprinkle on the flour and cook for 1 minute, stirring continuously. Gradually stir in the stock or water. Add the herbs and cook for 2 minutes.
4 Grind the nuts roughly and add along with the rice, egg and pepper.
5 Pack the mixture into a terrine or loaf tin, cover with foil and tuck the edges under to secure tightly.
6 Steam for 45 minutes above a pan of boiling water or pressure cook for 15 minutes.

Vegetable and Fruit Kebabs with Orange and Ginger Sauce

Serves 4

If fresh sweetcorn is not available, use frozen. Use a carton of orange juice rather than fresh oranges as this is not quite as acidic and makes the sauce less sharp. Another vegetable could be substituted for the mushrooms or sweetcorn, such as onion or tomatoes, and cubes of chicken or lamb could be used instead of the bananas. For extra flavour, add 30ml/2 tbsp of shoyu/tamari sauce (if your diet allows). This will also enable water to be used instead of the stock.

KEBABS	SAUCE
2 corn on the cob	140ml/5 fl oz/⅔ cup orange juice
2 large courgettes (zucchini)	
1 red pepper	5ml/1 tsp grated orange rind
2 bananas	5ml/1 tsp grated ginger
8 medium mushrooms	20ml/2 dsp sunflower oil
4 large *or* 8 small skewers	5ml/1 tsp mustard
	pinch cayenne pepper
	black pepper
	2 cloves garlic
	285ml/10 fl oz/1⅓ cups good stock
	15ml/1 level tbsp corn flour (cornstarch)

1 Make a marinade by mixing all the sauce ingredients except the stock and corn flour (cornstarch).
2 Cut the sweetcorn, courgettes (zucchini), pepper and bananas into 8 pieces. Place all the vegetables and fruit into a Tupperware container with a tight-fitting lid. Pour over the marinade and allow to stand for at least 2 hours, turning the container occasionally to coat the vegetables.

3 Thread the kebab ingredients onto 4 large or 8 small skewers.
4 Place the kebabs on a baking tray, cover with foil and bake in the oven at 400°F/200°C/Gas Mark 6 for 30 minutes.
5 Pour the remaining marinade into a pan together with the stock and the corn flour (cornstarch). Mix until smooth and bring the sauce to the boil, stirring constantly. When the kebabs have cooked, pour any juices from the tray into the sauce.
6 Place the kebabs on a bed of rice and serve with the sauce poured over. Accompany with a crisp salad.

Vegetable Risotto

Serves 4

For extra flavour, add 15ml/1 tbsp finely sliced fresh ginger or, if acceptable, 15ml/1 tbsp shoyu/tamari sauce. To add interest, vary the vegetables (try green beans, mangetout, broccoli or cauliflower, for example), and use millet, buckwheat or quinoa instead of the rice. Try serving with Tomato Sauce *(see Chapter 8, page 204)*.

170g/6 oz/¾ cup brown rice	40ml/2 tbsp sweetcorn *or* frozen peas
2 carrots	
1 small parsnip	55g/2 oz/½ cup toasted slivered almonds
1 onion	
1 stick (stalk) celery	15ml/1 tbsp parsley
1 courgette (zucchini)	black pepper
10ml/1 dsp olive oil	90ml/3 fl oz/⅓ cup water
handful beansprouts	

1 Boil the rice until just cooked. Sieve and keep warm.
2 Peel the carrots and parsnips, then continue peeling using a vegetable peeler so that the vegetables form thin slivers.
3 Dice the onion and celery and slice the courgettes (zucchini).
4 Sweat the vegetables in the olive oil, starting with the onion and celery, then add the carrot, parsnip and courgette (zucchini).
5 Add the beansprouts and sweetcorn, then the almonds, rice, parsley, pepper and water. Mix well, heat through and simmer for 3 minutes or until the water has been absorbed.

Stir-Fried Vegetables with Toasted Cashews

Serves 4

Serve with plain boiled rice, millet or quinoa and a side salad.

For a variation, if allowed, dissolve 10ml/1 dsp light miso, 10ml/1 dsp tomato purée and 20ml/2 dsp shoyu/tamari sauce in 285ml/½ pt/1⅓ cups of boiling water. Use this instead of the stock. You will not need to add the corn flour (cornstarch) as this produces a delicious thickened sauce.

Choose 6 vegetables from the following:
1 onion
1 carrot
2 sticks (stalks) celery
½ pepper
2 courgettes (zucchini)
12 baby sweetcorn
16 sugar snap peas *or* mangetout
115g/4 oz/1 cup green beans
55g/2 oz/⅓ cup water chestnuts
115g/4 oz/1½ cups red *or* white cabbage

115g/4 oz/2 cups spinach
170g/6 oz/3 cups broccoli *or* cauliflower florets
115g/4 oz/1 cup mushrooms

15ml/1tbsp olive oil
285ml/½ pint/1⅓ cups good stock
15ml/1 level tbsp corn flour (cornstarch)
115g/4 oz/1 cup toasted cashews

1 Cut the vegetables into shapes that will cook in equal times.
2 Sweat the vegetables in the oil until they begin to soften and brown.
3 Add the stock, cover and cook for a few more minutes.
4 Mix the corn flour (cornstarch) to a smooth paste with a little water and add to the vegetables, stirring all the time. Bring to the boil and simmer until the mixture thickens.
5 Add the cashews and serve.

Brazilian Stir-Fry

Serves 4

The almonds need to be very finely ground to thicken the sauce, so shop-bought ones are best. To vary, add 140g/5 oz/¾ cup smoked tofu or cooked chicken instead of one of the vegetables.

55g/2 oz/⅓ cup creamed coconut	2 carrots
285ml/½ pint/1⅓ cups boiling water	2 sticks (stalks) celery
	8 broccoli florets
	55g/2 oz/½ cup green beans
	115g/4 oz/1 cup mushrooms
Select 6 of the following vegetables:	115g/4 oz/1½ cups white cabbage
2 onions	
8 cauliflower florets	15ml/1 tbsp olive oil
12 baby sweetcorn	55g/2 oz/⅔ cup ground almonds
2 courgettes (zucchini)	5ml/1 tsp grated fresh ginger
55g/2 oz/½ cup mangetout	3ml/½ tsp dried thyme
½ pepper	black pepper

1 Dissolve the creamed coconut in the boiling water.
2 Cut the vegetables into pieces that will cook in equal times.
3 Sweat the vegetables in the oil until they all are just cooked.
4 Add the coconut water, the ground almonds, the ginger, the thyme and some black pepper. Heat through and serve with rice, millet or another starchy side dish.

Broccoli and Sweetcorn Quiche

Serves 4

Cabbage leaves are used instead of pastry in this quiche. Other ingredients could be used to make quiches, such as tuna fish, prawns, cubed smoked tofu, spinach, mushrooms, courgettes (zucchini) and peppers.

If you cannot eat eggs, try using 425g/15 oz/1½ cups of silken tofu and 260ml/9 fl oz/1¼ cups of soya milk instead of the eggs and milk. The flan will set but will not rise as it would when using eggs.

6–8 large cabbage leaves	425ml/¾ pint/2 cups soya *or* almond milk
455g/1 lb/8 cups broccoli florets	
2 large onions	black pepper
10ml/1 dsp olive oil	225g/8 oz/1 cup sweetcorn kernels
15ml/1 tbsp fresh parsley	
3 eggs	55g/2 oz/⅔ cup ground nuts

1 Cook the cabbage and the broccoli in boiling water for approximately 5 minutes until the cabbage leaves are soft enough to line the dish and the broccoli is still crunchy.
2 Cool the broccoli quickly by dipping in cold water to prevent over-cooking.
3 Chop the onions and sweat in the oil until they begin to brown and soften. Mix in the parsley.
4 Beat the eggs and milk and season with black pepper.
5 Use the cabbage leaves to double-line a deep 25-cm/10-inch quiche dish.
6 Scatter half the onions over the base, then arrange the broccoli florets making sure they do not come above the top of the dish.
7 Fill the gaps between the broccoli with sweetcorn, then scatter over the remaining onions. The dish should be packed with vegetables.
8 Pour over the egg and milk mixture and scatter the ground nuts over the surface.
9 Bake at 400°F/200°C/Gas Mark 6 for approximately 40–50 minutes or until the centre of the quiche is just setting. Do not overcook or the eggs will start to curdle and spoil the quiche.

Carrot and Leek Quiche

Serves 4

If you do not want to use tuna fish or tofu, substitute another vegetable such as green beans, red kidney beans or courgettes (zucchini). If you cannot eat eggs, try using 425g/15 oz/1½ cups of silken tofu and 260ml/9 fl oz/1¼ cups of soya milk instead of the eggs and milk. The quiche will set but will not rise as it would when using eggs.

FOR THE BASE:
1 quantity Rice Pancake Mixture
(see page 126

565g/1¼ lb/5 cups leeks, sliced
15ml/1 tbsp fresh parsley
3 eggs
425ml/¾ pint/2 cups soya milk
black pepper
2 medium carrots, grated
200g/7 oz/1⅓ cups smoked tofu
or tuna fish
55g/2 oz/⅔ cup ground nuts

1 Make 4 pancakes using the rice pancake mixture and use to line a greased, deep, 25-cm/10-inch flan dish.
2 Cook the leeks in a little water until they are almost tender. Drain well and mix in the parsley.
3 Beat the eggs with the milk and season with black pepper.
4 Layer half the carrots and leeks in the flan dish and cover with the cubed tofu or drained tuna fish. Repeat with a second layer of carrots and leeks.
5 Pour over the eggs and milk, then sprinkle with the ground nuts.
6 Bake for 40–50 minutes at 400°F/200°C/Gas Mark 6 until the centre of the flan is just setting. Do not overcook or the eggs will start to curdle.

Potato, Courgette (Zucchini) and Aubergine (Eggplant) Bake

Serves 4

If possible, use a food processor to slice the potatoes as this means they will be finely sliced and will cook easily. Tuna fish makes a good substitute for the olives, and sun-dried tomatoes and mushrooms could be used instead of the spinach. Note that the only acceptable sun-dried tomatoes I have found are dried and need soaking to reconstitute. Use carrot juice if you cannot tolerate tomatoes. Serve with salads.

1¼ kg/2½ lb/8 cups potatoes	1 tin (400g/15 oz/2 cups)
2 onions	chopped tomatoes in juice
4 courgettes (zucchini)	5 ml/1 tsp dried oregano
1 aubergine (eggplant)	6 sun-dried tomatoes
455g/1 lb/8 cups spinach	10 olives, halved
black pepper	olive oil

1 Finely slice the potatoes and the onion, then cut the courgettes (zucchini) and the aubergine (eggplant) into 2-cm/½-inch slices. Lightly cook the spinach in the water which remains on the leaves after washing.
2 Layer half the potatoes in a large, greased gratin dish or roasting tin. Season with black pepper.
3 Place half the sliced onions on top, then all the aubergine (eggplant) and courgette (zucchini) slices. Season with black pepper.
4 Mix the tinned tomatoes with the oregano and spread on top of the vegetables.
5 Sprinkle the chopped sun-dried tomatoes and the olives over the surface.
6 Cover with a layer of spinach, then the remaining onions and the potatoes.
7 Brush the surface with olive oil and bake in the centre of the oven at 400°F/200°C/Gas Mark 6 for 1¼ hours. Cover with foil if the potatoes start to brown too much.

Polenta Pizza

Serves 4

The base will remain soft and will need careful handling when serving. Serve along with a selection of salads. Add a few slivers of goat's cheese to the topping, if allowed.

115g/4 oz/⅔ cup polenta flour *or* maize meal 570ml/1 pint/2½ cups water 15ml/1 tbsp olive oil 3 ml/½ tsp dried oregano 40ml/2 rounded tbsp tomato purée Toppings to choose from: sliced peppers sliced spring onions (scallions) sweetcorn kernels sliced mushrooms black *or* green olives	pine nuts tuna fish sardines finely sliced onion sliced tomatoes artichoke hearts sliced courgettes (zucchini) sun-dried tomatoes pineapple prawns garlic olive oil for dribbling on the surface

1 Mix the polenta flour or maize meal with 140ml/½ pt/⅔ cup cold water in a pan (preferably non-stick). Add 425ml/¾ pint/2 cups of boiling water, mixing as you add.
2 Bring to the boil and simmer over a low heat, stirring constantly for 5 minutes. The mixture should be thick and smooth. Beat in the olive oil.
3 Grease a 30-cm/10–12-inch pizza pan or similar sized baking tray, and spread the hot mixture over the surface to form a pizza base.
4 Spread the tomato purée on top and sprinkle with oregano.
5 Add the toppings of your choice, making sure you build up a substantial layer.
6 Drizzle the surface with olive oil and bake in a preheated oven at 400°F/200°C/Gas Mark6 for 30–35 minutes.

Onion and Herb Bread Pizza

Serves 4

Use the ingredients for Onion and Herb Loaf *(see Chapter 9, page 221)* to make the pizza base. The flavourings can be omitted if you prefer a plain base. Bake for 10 minutes, then remove the base from the oven. Spread tomato purée and oregano over the surface, then add your chosen topping *(see previous recipe)*. Return to the oven and bake for a further 10–15 minutes or until the base is brown around the edges and the topping is cooked.

Vegetable Lasagne

Serves 4

If you cannot tolerate corn, try using cooked rice pancakes *(see page 126)* instead of the Polenta Lasagne. Those who can eat cheese could sprinkle a little on the surface before cooking.

LASAGNE:
115g/4 oz/⅔ cup polenta flour
or maize meal
570ml/1 pint/2½ cups water
15ml/1 tbsp olive oil

FILLING
3 onions
2 courgettes (zucchini)
2 sticks (stalks) celery
1 carrot
6 sun-dried tomatoes
10ml/1 dsp olive oil
3ml/½ tsp dried oregano
3ml/½ tsp dried basil
30ml/2 tbsp tomato purée
60ml/2 fl oz/¼ cup water
10 black olives

WHITE SAUCE:
30ml/2 level tbsp corn flour (cornstarch)
5ml/1 tsp mustard
425ml/¾ pint/2 cups soya *or* almond milk
black pepper
2ml/¼ tsp nutmeg

1 Mix the polenta flour with 140ml/¼ pint/½ cup of cold water in a pan. Add 425ml/¾ pint/2 cups of boiling water, mixing as you add. Bring to the boil and cook for 5 minutes, stirring constantly. Add the olive oil and mix well.

2 Grease a baking tray twice the size of the dish you intend to use for the lasagne. Spread the polenta onto the baking tray making a thin sheet. Allow to cool and cut in half, then use the sheets of polenta instead of lasagne.

3 To make the filling, dice the onions, courgettes (zucchini), celery and carrot and chop the sun-dried tomatoes. Sweat the vegetables in the olive oil until they begin to soften. Add the remaining filling ingredients and mix well.

4 To make the white sauce, mix the corn flour (cornstarch) with the mustard and a little milk in a saucepan until smooth. Add the remaining sauce ingredients and bring to the boil, stirring constantly.

5 To assemble the lasagne, place half the vegetable mixture into a gratin or lasagne dish and cover with a sheet of polenta. Repeat with the remaining vegetables and polenta. Pour the white sauce over the surface.

6 Bake for approximately 40 minutes at 400°F/200°C/Gas Mark 6.

Seafood Lasagne

Use tuna fish and prawns instead of the olives and sun-dried tomatoes in the above recipe.

Lentil Lasagne

Use the Lentil Bolognese recipe *(see page 121)* instead of the vegetable mixture in the above recipe.

Stuffed Baked Potatoes

Serves 4

> 4 large baking potatoes | filling *(see below)*

1 Wash the potatoes and prick the skins to prevent bursting.
2 Bake for 1¼ hours in the centre of the oven at 400°F/200°C/Gas Mark 6.
3 When cooked, split the potatoes in half and mash by pressing a fork into the flesh. Pile one of the following fillings into the centre.

Mushroom and Tomato Filling

Sauté 170g/6 oz/2 cups of sliced mushrooms in a little oil, add the diced flesh of 4 skinned tomatoes and 12 quartered olives. Heat through but do not cook or the tomatoes will become too soft.

Tuna, Celery and Egg or Avocado Filling

Mix a tin of drained tuna fish (200g/7 oz/1⅓ cups) with 2 diced hardboiled eggs (or 1 avocado), 2 large sticks (stalks) of celery diced and 80ml/4 tbsp mayonnaise.

Tahini and Tomato Filling

Scoop the flesh out of the potatoes and mash in a bowl. Add 60ml/4 tbsp of tahini, the flesh of 4 tomatoes skinned and diced and 10ml/1 dsp of tomato purée and mix to combine. Pile back into the potato shells and sprinkle the surface with sunflower seeds.

Chicken or Butterbean in White Sauce Filling

Make a White Sauce *(see Chapter 8, page 201)* and add 170g/6 oz/1¼ cups of cooked chicken (or cooked butter beans), 55g/2 oz/¼ cup of frozen peas and 15ml/1 tbsp of fresh chopped herbs, such as parsley, tarragon or coriander.

Prawns with Sweetcorn and Celery Filling

Mix 115g/4 oz/1 cup of prawns with 55g/2 oz/¼ cup of sweetcorn kernels or peas, 2 large sticks (stalks) of celery diced and 80ml/4 rounded tbsp of mayonnaise.

Other fillings which could be used include houmous *(see Chapter 2, page 77)*, ratatouille *(see Chapter 8, page 203)*, Lentil Bolognese *(see page 121)*, Avocado and Cashew Nut Pâté *(see Chapter 2, page 74)*, coleslaw *(see Chapter 4, page 109)*, Tropical Curried Chicken Salad *(see Chapter 4, page 117)*, or Minted Avocado and Chickpea Salad *(see Chapter 4, page 110)*.

Winter Bean and Tofu Casserole

Serves 4

This is a delicious casserole for a cold winter's day. Serve it along with rice, millet, quinoa or baked potatoes and a salad, or crusty garlic bread, if your diet allows. Omit the tofu if not tolerated and substitute another vegetable or different beans. For extra flavour, 15ml/1 tbsp of shoyu/tamari sauce can be added.

1 whole corn on the cob	3ml/½ tsp dried thyme
½ small swede	3ml/½ tsp dried rosemary
1 large parsnip	1 bay leaf
2 medium onions	black pepper
2 carrots	425ml/15 fl oz/2 cups water
2 courgettes (zucchini)	285ml/10 fl oz/1⅓ cups soya *or*
170g/6 oz/1 cup plain tofu	almond milk
225g/8 oz/1⅓ cups cooked red	30ml/2 level tbsp corn flour
kidney beans	(cornstarch)

1 Cut the corn on the cob into 2-cm/½-inch sections.
2 Cut the vegetables into chunks, adjusting the size according to how quickly they will cook. Place all the vegetables into a casserole dish.
3 Cube the tofu and add to the casserole along with the kidney beans, herbs, pepper and water. Mix gently.
4 Cover the casserole and cook for 1 hour at 400°F/200°C/Gas Mark 6. There should be only a small amount of liquid left in the casserole once cooked but watch to make sure it does not dry up altogether.
5 When cooked, lift out the vegetables and tofu using a slotted spoon, and remove the bay leaf.
6 Mix the soya or almond milk to a smooth paste with the corn flour (cornstarch) and add to the juices in the casserole dish. Bring to the boil on top of the cooker, stirring constantly, and simmer for 2 minutes. Return the vegetables to the pan and gently mix.

Bean and Vegetable Casserole

Serves 4

Serve with rice, millet, quinoa or baked potatoes and a salad. A variety of casseroles can be made by substituting other ingredients. Use carrot juice or other vegetable juice instead of the tomatoes. Use other herbs, such as 5ml/1 tsp of dill seeds, 5ml/1 tsp of fennel and 3ml/½ tsp of marjoram. Substitute other vegetables, such as peppers, leeks, fennel, cauliflower, kohlrabi, turnip and celeriac. Buckwheat could be used instead of the beans – cook the buckwheat first for 12 minutes, then drain and add to the casserole. Extra flavour can be added for those allowed by including 5ml/1 tsp of miso or 15ml/1 tbsp of shoyu/tamari sauce.

55g/2 oz/⅓ cup red split lentils	1 onion
1 tin (400g/15 oz/2 cups chopped tomatoes in juice	1 large carrot
	1 parsnip
1 clove garlic	2 sticks (stalks) celery
5ml/1 tsp grated ginger	2 courgettes (zucchini)
5ml/1 tsp paprika	115g/4 oz/1 cup green beans
5ml/1 tsp ground cumin	8 broccoli florets
5ml/1 tsp ground coriander	170g/6 oz/1 cup cooked beans
black pepper	(chickpeas, black eye, kidney, etc)
1 bay leaf	285ml/½ pt/1⅓ cups water

1 Place the lentils, the tomatoes, the pressed garlic clove, the ginger, the herbs and the spices in a casserole dish and mix.
2 Cut the vegetables into chunks. Vary the size according to how quickly they cook. Place on top of the lentil mix along with the beans.
3 Pour the water over the ingredients but do not mix at this stage. The lentils need to stay at the bottom of the casserole in the liquid in order to cook.
4 Cover the casserole and bake in the centre of the oven at 400°F/ 200°C/Gas Mark 6 for 1 hour, mixing gently half-way through. Remove the bay leaf before serving.

Broccoli and Smoked Tofu Bake

Serves 4

If tofu is not tolerated, try substituting tuna fish, cooked chicken, chopped hardboiled eggs or another vegetable instead.

1 medium onion	TOPPING:
225g/8 oz/4 cups broccoli florets	85g/3 oz/1 cup millet flakes
30ml/2 level tbsp rice flour	30g/1 oz/⅙ cup brown rice flour
285ml/½ pt/1⅓ cups soya milk	55g/2 oz/⅔ cup ground nuts,
2ml/¼ tsp nutmeg	e.g. almonds, hazelnuts
3ml/½ tsp lemon rind	20ml/2 dsp sunflower oil
black pepper	30ml/2 tbsp sunflower seeds
225g/8 oz/1½ cups cooked red kidney beans	
225g/8 oz/1¼ cups smoked tofu	

1 Chop the onion and cook with the broccoli in 140ml/¼ pt/⅔ cup of boiling water until just tender. Drain and reserve the cooking liquid.
2 Place the rice flour in a pan and mix to a smooth paste using a little soya milk. Add the remaining soya milk and the stock from the vegetables made up to 140ml/¼ pt/⅔ cup with water.
3 Bring to the boil, stirring constantly, then lower the heat and simmer for 2 minutes.
4 Add the nutmeg, lemon rind and pepper, then the vegetables, beans and the tofu which should be cubed.
5 Spoon the mixture into a large gratin dish (or 4 small dishes).
6 To make the topping, place the millet flakes, rice flour and ground nuts in a bowl and rub in the oil by hand.
7 Spread the topping over the vegetable and tofu mixture and scatter the sunflower seeds over the surface.
8 Bake for 15 minutes or until the topping is brown at 400°F/200°C/Gas Mark 6 on the top shelf of the oven.

Vegetable Crumble

Serves 4

Follow the previous recipe but substitute a 680g/1½lb/6–8 cups selection of vegetables instead of the tofu and kidney beans – try leeks, parsnips, carrots, celery, courgettes (zucchini), etc. Cook all the vegetables together in just over 140ml/¼ pt/⅔ cup of water and add 3ml/½ tsp of dried rosemary and 3ml/½ tsp of dried thyme to the sauce. Keep the remaining ingredients the same and cook for 15 minutes, as before.

Vegetable and Cashew Nut Medley

Serves 4

Serve in individual gratin dishes or as a sauce to go with rice or pasta. Accompany with salads.

Other vegetables which substitute well in this dish include onions, baby sweetcorn, water chestnuts, mangetout or sugar snap peas. Try walnuts or toasted slivered almonds instead of the cashews. If it is tolerated, add 15ml/1 tbsp of shoyu/tamari sauce to the sauce ingredients.

85g/3 oz/¾ cup green beans
1 courgette (zucchini)
1–2 sticks (stalks) celery
½ red pepper
1 leek
1 medium carrot
115g/4 oz/1 cup whole cashews
170g/6 oz/3 cups broccoli florets

SAUCE:
5ml/1 tsp tomato purée
5ml/1 tsp grated ginger
10ml/1 dsp lemon juice
3ml/½ tsp grated lemon rind
30ml/2 tbsp orange juice
2ml/¼ tsp nutmeg
5ml/1 tsp paprika
15ml/1 tbsp fresh coriander
15ml/1 tbsp corn flour (cornstarch)
340ml/12 fl oz/1½ cups stock
(use vegetable cooking liquid and water)

1 Cut the beans in half and slice the courgette (zucchini), celery, red pepper and leek. Cut the carrot into matchstick pieces. Toast the cashews.
2 Place the vegetables in a pan with 285ml/10 fl oz/1⅓ cups of boiling water. Bring to the boil and simmer for 5 minutes or until the vegetables are just cooked but slightly crisp. Drain, keeping the liquid for stock.
3 To make the sauce, place all the sauce ingredients except the stock in a pan and mix to a smooth paste. Add the stock gradually.
4 Bring to the boil, stirring constantly, and simmer for 2 minutes. Add the vegetables and cashew nuts to the sauce and allow to heat through.

Potato and Parsnip Pie Crust

Potatoes and parsnips are used to make a pie crust which can then be filled with one of the following fillings or one of your choice.

455g/1 lb/3½ cups potatoes	black pepper
340g/12 oz/2⅓ cups parsnips	olive oil for brushing

1 Cut the potatoes and parsnips into equal sized chunks and cook together in boiling water until tender.
2 Sieve, and save the cooking liquid.
3 Mash the potatoes and the parsnips with some black pepper and sufficient cooking liquid to make them soft and smooth.
4 Press into a greased 23-cm/9-in pie dish, moulding with the fingers to form a pie shape. Brush the surface with olive oil and bake in the oven for 45 minutes at 400°F/200°C/Gas Mark 6.

Spinach and Egg Filling

Serves 4

4 hardboiled eggs	425ml/¾ pint/2 cups White
455g/1 lb/8 cups spinach	Sauce *(see Chapter 8, page 201)*
	paprika

1 Halve the hardboiled eggs and lay cut side down into the pie.
2 Shred the spinach and then cook in the water in which it has been washed for no more than 5 minutes or until it is soft and wilted. Drain and spread over the eggs.
3 Make the White Sauce as directed and pour over the eggs and spinach. Sprinkle with paprika and serve.

Fennel, Lentil and Almond Filling

Serves 4

Cut 2 bulbs of fennel into quarters. Steam until just tender. Cover with dahl sauce *(see page 206)* and sprinkle with 30g (1oz/¼ cup) toasted, slivered almonds.

Leek, Courgette and Mushroom Filling

Serves 4

225g/8oz/2 cups leeks (mainly white stems)	10ml/1 dsp olive oil
340g/12oz/3 cups courgettes	10 black olives
225g/8oz/2¾ cups mushrooms	4 sundried tomatoes
	black pepper

1 Slice the leeks and courgettes and cut the mushrooms in halves or quarters. Cut the olives in half and dice the sundried tomatoes.
2 Sweat the leeks for a few minutes then add the courgettes and the mushrooms, sweat until cooked. Mix in the olives and sundried tomatoes and season with black pepper. Pile into the pie crust and serve.

Stuffed Peppers

Serves 4

Serve as a vegetarian main course with potatoes and salad or as a vegetable accompaniment. The peppers could also be stuffed with Nut Roast *(see page 131)* or Millet and Walnut Bake *(see page 124)* ingredients.

1 onion	55g/2 oz/¼ cup sweetcorn
1 clove garlic	kernels *or* frozen peas
10ml/1 dsp olive oil	10ml/1 dsp fresh chopped mint
225g/8 oz/1⅓ cups cooked rice	10ml/1 dsp fresh chopped
20ml/2 dsp raisins (optional)	parsley
30ml/2 tbsp pine nuts *or*	3ml/½ tsp ground cinnamon
cashew nuts	black pepper
	4 medium green or red peppers

1 Chop the onion and sweat along with the pressed clove of garlic in the olive oil until they begin to soften and brown.
2 Add all the remaining ingredients except the peppers and mix well.
3 Cut a circular hole in the top of each pepper, removing the stalk. Use a spoon to scoop out internal fibres and seeds.
4 Hold each of the peppers in turn over the pan containing the stuffing mixture. Using a spoon, fill each pepper with the mixture and press it down well.
5 Place the peppers in a deep-sided ovenproof dish. Cut a little off the base of the peppers, if necessary, to enable them to stand easily.
6 Pour 140ml/¼ pint/⅔ cup of water around the peppers and cover with foil. Bake in the centre of the oven at 400°F/200°C/Gas Mark 6 for 50–60 minutes or until the peppers are soft but not mushy.

Stuffed Aubergines (Eggplants)

Serves 4

Serve with salad and vegetables as a main course or individually as starters. Millet or quinoa could be used instead of the rice. The original recipe used 115g/4 oz/2 cups breadcrumbs instead of the rice and ground almonds. If permitted, try this for a variation. Half a tin of flaked tuna fish (100g/3½ oz/½ cup) or 30ml/2 tbsp grated cheese can be added for extra flavour, if allowed, and the olives could be omitted. Meat-eaters will begin to think vegetarian after eating this.

2 large aubergines (eggplants)	10ml/1 dsp fresh chopped parsley
1 onion	10ml/1 dsp fresh chopped coriander
1 clove garlic	black pepper
5ml/1 tsp olive oil	55g/2 oz/⅓ cup cooked rice
4 medium tomatoes	55g/2 oz/⅔ cup ground almonds
12 black olives	olive oil for drizzling on the surface
5ml/1 tsp tomato purée	
3ml/½ tsp dried marjoram	
3ml/½ tsp dried oregano	

1 Cut the aubergines (eggplants) in half and scoop out the flesh leaving 2cm/½ an inch around the edge next to the skin. Dice the flesh finely and place in a large bowl.
2 Finely dice the onion and press the garlic clove. Sweat the onion and garlic in 5ml/1 tsp of olive oil until they begin to soften and brown. Add these to the diced aubergine (eggplant) flesh in the bowl.
3 Skin the tomatoes and dice the flesh. Quarter the black olives. Add to the bowl along with the remaining ingredients and mix.
4 Place the aubergine (eggplant) shells on a baking tray, in a gratin dish or in individual dishes.
5 Pile the stuffing into the shells, pressing down firmly.
6 Drizzle the surface with olive oil, cover with foil and bake at 400°F/200°C/Gas Mark 6 for 1 hour or until the aubergines (eggplants) are quite soft.

Stuffed Marrow

Use the recipe for Stuffed Aubergines to make stuffed marrow. Peel the marrow, cut into 4-cm/1½-inch slices and remove the centres. The centres can be finely diced and added to the filling ingredients unless the marrows are old and full of seeds. If this is the case, use another length of marrow to chop up for the filling. Bake for approximately ½ hour.

Rice with Sweetcorn and Coconut

Serves 4

Serve as a side dish.

225g/8 oz/1¼ cups sweetcorn kernels *or* frozen peas	90ml/3 fl oz/⅓ cup boiling water
30g/1 oz/⅙ cup creamed coconut	30ml/3 dsp desiccated coconut
	225g/8 oz/1⅓ cups cooked rice

1 Break the sweetcorn kernels (or peas) in a bowl with a fork.
2 Dissolve the creamed coconut in the boiling water.
3 Add all the ingredients to a pan and bring slowly to the boil, stirring frequently.
4 Turn off the heat and leave to stand, covered, for 5 minutes.

Carrot and Coconut Rice

Serves 4

Serve as a side dish.

30g/1 oz/⅙ cup creamed coconut	3ml/½ tsp ground nutmeg
90ml/3 fl oz/⅓ cup boiling water	225g/8 oz/1⅓ cups cooked rice
5 cardamom pods *or* 3ml/½ tsp ground cardamom	225g/8 oz/1⅓ cups carrots, grated

1 Dissolve the creamed coconut in the boiling water. If using cardamom pods, split the pods and remove the seeds, throwing away the empty shells.
2 Place all the ingredients into a pan and bring slowly to the boil, stirring frequently.
3 Cover and simmer for 4–5 minutes, or until the carrots are cooked.

Sushi

| 2 sheets sushi nori (toasted dried seaweed) | 1 portion rice with sweetcorn *or* carrot and coconut rice |

1 Lay the sheets of nori on a flat surface and divide the rice between them. Spread the rice out, pressing it down and keeping it 3cm/1 inch away from the farthest and nearest edges.
2 Roll up the nori sheets like a Swiss roll, dampening the farthest edge so that it sticks to itself and seals the roll.
3 Allow to cool. Cut the sushi roll into 3-cm/1-inch slices to serve as snacks or cut into 8-cm/3-inch lengths to serve with vegetables or salads.

Indian Food

Indian food fits very well into this eating regime. It is an ideal way to entertain as a wide selection of dishes can be offered, most of which are allowed. Try the following four dishes but also include the Chicken Curry *(see page 165)*, the Spicy Baked Chicken *(see page 170)* or the Lamb Korma *(see page 176)* from Chapter 6. Add a few salads from Chapter 4 as curry accompaniments, such as Apple, Carrot and Ginger *(see page 108)*; Cucumber, Mint and Yogurt *(see page 107)* or Tomato and Coriander *(see page 107)* and some naan bread or poppadoms for those allowed wheat. With food like this, who would mind being on a special diet?

Vegetable Masala

Serves 4

680g/1½lb/6–8 cups selection of vegetables, such as: cauliflower florets leeks carrots broccoli celery onions courgettes (zucchini) parsnips green beans sweetcorn	15ml/1 tbsp olive oil 5ml/1 tsp garam masala 3ml/½ tsp ground cumin 3ml/½ tsp ground coriander 2ml/⅓ tsp ground cardamom 3ml/½ tsp fennel seeds 3ml/½ tsp turmeric 5ml/1 tsp paprika 55g/2 oz/⅓ cup creamed coconut 285ml/½ pt/1⅓ cups boiling water 15ml/1 tbsp lemon juice 5ml/1 tsp grated ginger 55g/2 oz/⅔ cup ground almonds

1 Cut the vegetables into shapes which will cook in roughly equal times. Sweat the vegetables in the olive oil until they begin to soften and brown.
2 Add the spices to the pan and sweat for another 2 minutes.
3 Dissolve the coconut in the boiling water and add to the vegetables along with the lemon juice, ginger and ground almonds. Stir to mix.
4 Simmer for another few minutes until all the vegetables are just cooked. Add a little more water if the mixture starts to become too dry. Serve with rice, millet or quinoa.

Biriani with Rice

Serves 4

Serve with plain boiled rice.

2 onions	5ml/1 tsp ground fennel
2 medium baking apples	3ml/½ tsp ground cardamom
1 clove garlic	5ml/1 tsp ground cumin
55g/2 oz/⅓ cup split red lentils	5ml/1 tsp ground coriander
55g/2 oz/⅓ cup creamed coconut	5ml/1 tsp turmeric
850ml/1½ pints/3¾ cups water	5ml/1 tsp garam masala
10ml/1 dsp tomato purée (optional)	5ml/1 tsp grated ginger
	55g/2 oz/⅔ cup ground almonds

1 Finely dice the onions, grate the baking apples and press the garlic clove. Wash the red lentils.
2 Place all the ingredients in a saucepan, bring to the boil and simmer gently for 30–40 minutes until the lentils disintegrate to form part of the sauce. Stir occasionally while cooking.

Quick Bean Curry

Serves 4

Use tinned beans for quickness, washing the beans well to remove the salt.

55g/2 oz/⅓ cup creamed coconut	1 tin (400g/15 oz/2 cups) chopped tomatoes in tomato juice
285ml/½ pt/1⅓ cups boiling water	1 clove garlic, pressed
½ pepper, diced	5ml/1 tsp grated ginger
85g/3 oz/⅓ cup sweetcorn *or* peas	5ml/1 tsp ground coriander
1 onion, diced	5ml/1 tsp ground cumin
225g/8 oz/1⅓ cups cooked beans (e.g. chickpeas, butterbeans)	15ml/1 tbsp fresh chopped coriander

1 Dissolve the coconut in the boiling water in a saucepan.
2 Add the remaining ingredients, bring to the boil and simmer for 15 minutes. Serve with rice, millet or quinoa.

Mushroom Curry

Add 340g/12 oz/3 cups of small button mushrooms instead of the beans to the previous recipe.

Vegetable Rogan Josh

Serves 4

I like to select just two or three vegetables and make, for instance, a cauliflower and courgette rogan josh or an okra, baby sweetcorn and fennel rogan josh. The variations are endless.

6 medium onions	3ml/½ tsp turmeric
2 cloves garlic	2ml/¼ tsp cardamom, ground *or*
15ml/1 tbsp olive oil	seeds
570ml/1 pint/2½ cups creamed	425ml/15 fl oz/2 cups water
tomatoes *or* tomato juice	5ml/1 tsp grated ginger
5ml/1 tsp ground coriander	680g/1½ lb/6–8 cups vegetables
5ml/1 tsp ground cumin	e.g. carrots, celery, peppers,
5ml/1 tsp fennel seeds	mushrooms, fennel, okra, baby
5ml/1 tsp garam masala	sweetcorn, broccoli, courgettes
5ml/1 tsp paprika	(zucchini)

1 Dice the onions and press the garlic cloves. Sweat the onions and garlic gently in the olive oil until they are a golden brown colour. This will take at least ½ hour. Do not rush, do not turn the heat up too high and stir frequently.
2 Blend half of the onions with half of the tomato juice in a food processor until they are smooth and creamy.
3 Add the spices to the pan with the remaining onions, and continue to sweat for 2–3 minutes, stirring constantly.
4 Add the water, the ginger and the vegetables cut into chunks. Stir to mix.
5 Bring to the boil and simmer for 10 minutes or until the vegetables are nearly cooked.
6 Add the tomato and onion mixture and the remaining tomato juice. Simmer for a further 5–10 minutes or until the vegetables are cooked. Serve with rice, millet or quinoa.

MeatDishesMeatDishesMeatDishes

Chicken Polo

Serves 4

2 onions	1 cinnamon stick *or* 3ml/½ tsp
1 clove garlic	ground cinnamon
1 large carrot	black pepper
55g/2 oz/¼ cup dried apricots	1 bay leaf
10ml/1 dsp olive oil	30ml/1 heaped tbsp raisins
225g/8 oz/1⅓ cups chicken	(optional)
breasts, diced	710ml/1¼ pints/3¼ cups stock
285g/10 oz/1⅓ cups short-grain	*or* water
rice	55g/2 oz/½ cup split almonds

1 Chop the onion, press the garlic and cut the carrot into matchstick pieces. Cut the apricots into small pieces.
2 Sweat the onion and the garlic in the oil until they begin to brown. Use a heavy-bottomed pan with a good-fitting lid.
3 Add the chicken and sauté for a few minutes until it starts to brown. Wash the rice well and add, along with the remaining ingredients (except the almonds).
4 Bring to the boil and simmer gently for 50–60 minutes until the rice is cooked. A little more water or stock may be needed near to the end of the cooking time to prevent the mixture sticking to the pan. The rice should be creamy and sticky when cooked.
5 Toast the almonds and stir in just before serving.

Chicken Curry

Serves 4

1 large onion
1 stick (stalk) celery
¼ green pepper
¼ red pepper
225g/8 oz/1⅓ cup cooked chicken
1 large baking apple
1 clove garlic
5ml/1 tsp hot madras curry powder

570ml/1 pint/2½ cups water *or* stock
15ml/1 tbsp desiccated coconut
15ml/1 tbsp tomato purée, optional
black pepper
10ml/1 level dsp corn flour (cornstarch)

1 Dice the onion, celery, peppers and the chicken and grate the baking apple. Press the garlic clove.
2 Place all the ingredients except the corn flour (cornstarch) into a saucepan, bring to the boil and simmer for 50 minutes, stirring occasionally.
3 Mix the corn flour (cornstarch) in a little water and stir into the curry to thicken. Reheat and cook for 2 minutes before serving.

Chicken Brazilian

Serves 4

3–4 chicken breasts	55g/2 oz/⅓ cup creamed coconut
15ml/1 tbsp lemon juice	
15ml/1 tbsp olive oil	140ml/¼ pt/⅔ cup boiling water
2 onions	2 large tomatoes
2 cloves garlic	55g/2 oz/⅔ cup ground almonds
1 green pepper	black pepper
	15ml/1 tbsp parsley

1 Cube the chicken, toss in the lemon juice and sweat in the olive oil until beginning to brown.
2 Chop the onions, press the garlic cloves and add to the chicken. Sweat for a further 5 minutes.
3 Slice the green pepper, dissolve the creamed coconut in the boiling water and skin and chop the tomatoes. Add to the pan along with the ground almonds and black pepper.
4 Stir, bring to the boil and simmer for 15 minutes, adding a little more liquid if the mixture starts to become too dry.
5 Add the parsley and serve with plain boiled rice, millet or quinoa.

Chicken Casserole

Serves 4

1 onion	10ml/1 dsp tomato purée
1 stick (stalk) celery	(optional)
2 carrots	3ml/½ tsp dried marjoram
1 clove garlic	3ml/½ tsp dried rosemary
1 dsp olive oil	2ml/¼ tsp dried sage
55g/2 oz/½ cup mushrooms	3ml/½ tsp paprika
(optional)	1 bay leaf
¼ green pepper	black pepper
285ml/½ pint/1⅓ cups water	4 chicken joints (skinned)
	5ml/1 tsp corn flour (cornstarch)

1 Cut the vegetables into bite-sized pieces and press the garlic clove. Sweat the onion, celery, carrots and garlic in the olive oil until beginning to soften and brown. Add the mushrooms and peppers and sweat for another few minutes.
2 Mix together the water, tomato purée, herbs and seasoning and pour over the vegetables.
3 Add the chicken pieces, cover the casserole and cook at 400°F/200°C/Gas Mark 6 for approximately 1¼ hours or until the chicken is tender.
4 Stir the corn flour (cornstarch) in a little water and add to the casserole to thicken it. Reheat and remove the bay leaf.
5 Serve with rice and a green salad or fresh vegetables.

Stir-Fried Chicken and Vegetables

Serves 4

An alternative sauce can be made, for those whose diets allow, by mixing 10ml/1 dsp tomato purée, 10ml/1 dsp light miso and 20ml/2 dsp shoyu/tamari with 285ml/½ pint/1⅓ cups of water. Add this instead of the stock and corn flour (cornstarch).

Select 3–4 vegetables from the following:
2 courgettes (zucchini)
115g/4 oz/1 cup mangetout
115g/4 oz/⅓ cup water chestnuts
115g/4 oz/2 cups broccoli florets
1 onion, sliced
½ red pepper
2 carrots

8 baby sweetcorn
55g/2 oz/½ cup mushrooms

1 clove garlic, pressed
15ml/1 tbsp olive oil
2 chicken breasts
285ml/½ pt/1⅓ cups stock *or* water
10ml/1 dsp corn flour (cornstarch)
black pepper

1 Cut the vegetables into pieces that will cook in approximately the same amount of time.
2 Sweat the vegetables and garlic in the olive oil for a few minutes. Add the chicken and sweat for 5 minutes.
3 Mix the stock to a smooth paste with the corn flour (cornstarch), and add to the vegetables and meat.
4 Bring to the boil and simmer for approximately 5 minutes until the vegetables and chicken are cooked.
5 Season with black pepper and serve with boiled rice and salads.

Chicken with Barbecue Sauce

Serves 4

30ml/2 tbsp lemon juice
30ml/2 tbsp tomato purée
5ml/1 tsp Chinese five spice powder
1 clove garlic, pressed
140ml/¼ pint/⅔ cup apple juice

140ml/¼ pint/⅔ cup stock *or* water
4 chicken breasts
10ml/1 dsp corn flour (cornstarch)

1 Mix all the ingredients except the chicken and the corn flour (cornstarch) to form a smooth sauce. Marinade the chicken in the sauce for at least 2 hours.
2 Remove the chicken from the marinade, place on a greased baking tray in the centre of the oven at 400°F/200°C/Gas Mark 6 for 30 minutes. Baste with the juices from the chicken once during cooking.
3 Mix the corn flour (cornstarch) to a smooth paste in a pan with a little of the marinade. Add the remaining marinade and any juices from the cooked chicken. Bring to the boil, stirring constantly, and allow to simmer for 2 minutes.
4 Serve the chicken on a bed of rice with the sauce poured over.

Spicy Baked Chicken

Serves 4

If your diet allows, add a little yogurt to any cooking juices from the chicken and serve as an accompaniment. Use foil to cover the baking tray to make washing-up easier.

2 cloves garlic	2ml/¼ tsp cayenne pepper
60ml/4 tbsp lemon juice	10ml/1 dsp turmeric
2ml/¼ tsp black pepper	4 chicken breasts *or* chicken
10ml/1 level dsp paprika	portions, skinned
10ml/1 level dsp ground cumin	parsley to garnish

1 Combine all the ingredients except the chicken. Rub the spice mixture into the chicken pieces and leave to marinade for at least 3 hours in a covered container.
2 Place the chicken pieces on a baking tray, cover with foil and bake in the centre of the oven at 400°F/200°C/Gas Mark 6 for 30 minutes if using chicken breasts and 1 hour if using joints.
3 Serve sprinkled with parsley, accompanied by brown rice and dahl *(see Chapter 8, page 206)* and with a salad or fresh vegetables.

Sima's Chicken

Serves 4

Omit the raisins if you cannot tolerate dried fruit.

225g/8 oz/1 cup brown rice	juice of 1 orange
340g/12 oz/2¼ cups cooked chicken	60ml/3 tbsp raisins (optional)
	black pepper
2 carrots	115g/4 oz/1¼ cups toasted
rind of ½ orange	flaked almonds

1　Cook the brown rice and keep warm.
2　Cut the chicken into bite-sized pieces or into small joints.
3　Cut the carrots into matchstick pieces. Thinly pare the orange rind and cut into matchstick strips.
4　Cook the carrots in the orange juice with the orange rind and raisins for appxorimately 5 minutes until just cooked. Warm the chicken.
5　Mix together the rice, the chicken, the carrot mixture (including any remaining cooking liquid), the black pepper and the nuts, and serve.

Chicken Liver Risotto

Serves 4

If you cannot use mushrooms, try substituting two finely sliced courgettes (zucchini). Use organic chicken livers, if possible.

225g/8 oz/1 cup brown rice	15ml/1 tbsp olive oil
3 medium onions	black pepper
225g/8 oz/2 cups mushrooms	3ml/½ tsp dried basil
225g/8 oz/1 cup chicken livers	

1 Cook the rice and keep warm.
2 Chop the onions, slice the mushrooms and cut the chicken livers into small pieces.
3 In a large frying pan or wok, sweat the onions in the oil until they begin to soften and brown.
4 Turn the heat full on, add the mushrooms and stir-fry for 2 minutes.
5 Add the chicken livers, black pepper and basil, and stir-fry until the mixture begins to brown and the liver is just cooked. This will only take a few minutes.
6 Add the rice, mix well and serve with salad and vegetables.

Rabbit or Chicken with Prunes

Serves 4

Accompany with brown rice, millet or quinoa and with salads or vegetables.

8 whole prunes	10ml/1 dsp lemon juice
10ml/1 dsp paprika	1 carrot, cut into matchsticks
5ml/1 tsp dried sage	2 onions, chopped
5ml/1 tsp dried thyme	2 large sticks (stalks) celery,
2ml/¼ tsp chilli powder	sliced
4 rabbit *or* chicken portions	black pepper
10ml/1 dsp tomato purée	1 bay leaf
425ml/¾ pint/2 cups water *or*	10ml/1 dsp corn flour
stock (including liquid in which	(cornstarch)
prunes were soaked)	

1 Soak the prunes for 2–3 hours in water which has been brought to the boil.
2 Mix the paprika, sage, thyme and chilli. Skin the meat and toss in the spices until it is coated all over. Place in a casserole dish.
3 Mix the tomato purée with the stock and the lemon juice and add to the casserole along with the vegetables, prunes, pepper and bay leaf.
4 Cook slowly in the oven at 370°F/185°C/Gas Mark 4 for approximately 2 hours.
5 Mix the corn flour (cornstarch) with a little water and stir into the casserole. Bring to the boil and cook for 2 minutes before serving.

Lamb with Orange and Ginger Sauce

Serves 4

Serve with brown rice, millet or quinoa and vegetables or salads.

10ml/1 dsp tomato purée	2 cloves garlic, pressed
5ml/1 tsp grated ginger	285ml/½ pint/1⅓ cups water
3ml/½ tsp dried ginger	565g/1¼ lb/2½ cups cubed lean
2ml/¼ tsp black pepper	lamb
3ml/½ tsp turmeric	2 medium onions, diced
5ml/1 tsp paprika	10ml/1 dsp corn flour
juice of 1 orange	(cornstarch)
grated rind of 1 orange	

1 Combine the liquids and flavourings in a casserole dish until smooth and well mixed.
2 Add the cubes of lamb and the onions and mix again.
3 Cook in the centre of the oven at 400°F/200°C/Gas Mark 6 for approximately 1½ hours or until the meat is tender.
4 Mix the corn flour (cornstarch) with a little water and stir into the casserole. Bring to the boil and simmer for 2 minutes.

Lamb Kebabs

Serves 4

Serve with plain rice or Nut Pilau *(see Lamb with Nut Pilau, page 177)* and salads.

1 clove garlic, pressed	5ml/1 tsp paprika
15ml/1 tbsp lemon juice	1 onion
15ml/1 tbsp tomato purée	8 medium mushrooms *or* 1 large
30ml/2 tbsp olive oil	pepper
3ml/½ tsp ground ginger	565g/1¼ lb/2½ cups lean lamb
2ml/¼ tsp black pepper	

1 Mix all the ingredients except the lamb and vegetables to form a marinade. Cube the lamb and toss in the marinade. Leave to stand for at least 2 hours.
2 Cut the onion into quarters and separate each quarter into its layers (a large piece of onion will not cook in the time it takes to cook the meat). If using the pepper, cut into eight pieces.
3 Thread the meat, mushrooms or pepper and the onion layers onto 4 large skewers. Brush the vegetables with the marinade.
4 Place on a baking tray and bake at 400°F/200°C/Gas Mark 6 for 30 minutes, turning once during cooking.

Lamb Korma with Bananas

Serves 4

Serve with brown rice, millet or quinoa and with curry accompaniments, salads or vegetables. If your diet allows, stir 140ml/¼ pint/⅔ cup of yogurt gradually into the korma just before serving.

5 onions	10ml/1 dsp tomato purée (optional)
15ml/1 tbsp olive oil	55g/2 oz/⅓ cup creamed coconut
5ml/1 tsp ground coriander	425ml/¾ pint/2 cups boiling water
3ml/½ tsp ground cumin	565g/1¼ lb/2½ cups lean lamb, cubed
3ml/½ tsp ground cardamom	20ml/1 rounded tbsp raisins (optional)
2ml/¼ tsp ground cloves	2 bananas
2ml/¼ tsp cinnamon	
3ml/½ tsp turmeric	
2ml/¼ tsp black pepper	
5ml/1 tsp garam masala	
2 cloves garlic, pressed	
5ml/1 tsp grated ginger	

1 Finely slice 3 onions and sweat in the olive oil over a gentle heat, stirring regularly, until they are soft and golden brown. This will take approximately 30 minutes.
2 Add the spices and the garlic, and sweat for another few minutes.
3 Place the onion mixture, the ginger and the tomato purée in a food processor and blend until very smooth.
4 In a large casserole dish, dissolve the creamed coconut in the boiling water. Add the onion mixture and the meat and mix well.
5 Roughly chop the two remaining onions and add to the casserole dish, along with the raisins.
6 Place the casserole in the oven at 400°F/200°C/Gas Mark 6, and cook for 1½ hours or until the meat is tender.
7 Cut the bananas into 2-cm/½-inch lengths, and add to the casserole just before serving. They only need a few minutes to warm through.

Chicken Korma with Green Pepper

Serves 4

Follow the previous recipe, substituting chicken for the lamb, green pepper for the bananas, and use a large tin of chopped tomatoes in tomato juice instead of 285ml/½ pint/1⅓ cups of water. Slice the green pepper and add along with the other ingredients.

Lamb with Nut Pilau

Serves 4

Accompany with a salad or fresh vegetables.

225g/8 oz/1 cup brown rice	2ml/¼ tsp turmeric
1 medium onion	3ml/½ tsp cinnamon
2 cloves garlic	710ml/1¼ pints/3¼ cups good
10ml/1 dsp olive oil	stock
2ml/¼ tsp ground cardamom	30g/1 oz/⅕ cup raisins (optional)
5ml/1 tsp ground cumin	4 lamb chops
5ml/1 tsp ground coriander	55g/2 oz/⅓ cup toasted split
1ml/⅛ tsp chilli powder	almonds

1 Soak the rice in lots of warm water for 20 minutes. Rinse and drain.
2 Finely chop the onion and press the garlic clove. Sweat the onion and garlic in the olive oil until they begin to soften and brown.
3 Add the rice and the spices, and sweat for another few minutes.
4 Add the stock and the raisins, bring to the boil, cover and simmer for approximately 50–60 minutes until the rice is cooked and all the liquid has been absorbed. To prevent the rice becoming too dry it may be necessary to add a little more water during cooking, especially towards the end.
5 Grill the chops while the rice is cooking.
6 Finally, toss the almonds into the rice, and serve with the chops.

FishDishesFishDishesFishDishes

ishDishesFishDishes FishDishes

Cod Provençale

This fish dish is quick and easy to make yet delicious enough for entertaining. Try salmon or monkfish instead of the cod or add prawns or mussels. If you cannot tolerate tomatoes, try using carrot juice.

3ml/½ tsp dried oregano	1 onion, chopped
3ml/½ tsp dried basil	1 green pepper, diced
2ml/¼ tsp dried thyme	1 clove garlic, pressed
5ml/1 tsp fennel seeds	455g/1 lb/2⅓ cups cod (thick
1 bay leaf	piece), cut *or* flaked into bite-
black pepper	sized pieces
140ml/5 fl oz/⅔ cup water	parsley to garnish
570ml/1 pint/2½ cups creamed	
tomatoes *or* tomato juice	

1 Place the herbs, seasoning, water, tomatoes, vegetables and garlic in a pan and cook for 10 minutes.
2 Add the fish to the tomato mixture and cook gently for 5 minutes or until the fish is just cooked. Do not stir roughly or the fish will break up.
3 Serve on rice, sprinkled with lots of fresh parsley.

Fish Florentine

Serves 4

You could bake the fish pieces together in a larger gratin dish, but extend the cooking time to approximately 20–25 minutes. A little grated cheese mixed with breadcrumbs could be used instead of the ground nuts, if your diet allows.

455g/1 lb/8 cups spinach	425ml/¾ pint/2 cups White
4 pieces fish e.g. cod, haddock,	Sauce *(see Chapter 8, page 201)*
salmon	20ml/2 dsp ground nuts

1 Wash the spinach and lightly cook in the water which remains on the leaves after washing, for 3–5 minutes.
2 Drain the spinach and divide between four individual gratin dishes.
3 Lay a piece of fish on each spinach bed.
4 Make the white sauce as directed and pour evenly over the fish. Sprinkle the nuts over the surface.
5 Bake for approximately 15 minutes near the top of the oven at 400°F/200°C/Gas Mark 6 until the top is lightly brown and the fish is just cooked.

Mackerel in Ginger and Orange

Serves 4

juice of 2 oranges	10ml/1 dsp tomato purée
grated rind of 1 orange	black pepper
5ml/1 tsp grated ginger	4 mackerel fillets

1 Mix together the orange juice, rind, ginger, tomato purée and pepper.
2 Marinate the mackerel fillets in the mixture for at least 3 hours.
3 Bake in a covered container in the marinade at 400°F/200°C/Gas Mark 6 for 20–25 minutes or until the fish is just cooked. Serve hot or cold with the juices poured over the fish.

Stir-Fry with Prawns and Peaches

Serves 4

If allowed, add 15ml/1tbsp of shoyu/tamari sauce for extra flavour. Note that prawns do contain salt unless freshly shelled.

1 bunch spring onions (scallions)	60ml/2 fl oz/¼ cup water
2 carrots	115g/4 oz/1 cup prawns
2 medium peaches	115g/4 oz/1 cup toasted
10ml/1 dsp olive oil	cashews
455g/1 lb/2⅔ cups cooked rice	black pepper

1 Finely slice the spring onions (scallions), cut the carrots into match-stick pieces and dice the peaches.
2 Sweat the carrots and spring onions (scallions) in the olive oil until just beginning to soften.
3 Add the remaining ingredients and sweat until the mixture is warmed through and the water has been absorbed.

Peppered Cod

Serves 4

Serve with crisp stir-fried vegetables, rice and salad. Green peppercorns are available bottled in brine. You could, however, use dried green or black peppercorns soaked overnight in a little boiling water, or even coarsely ground black pepper. Use dried herbs if you do not have fresh or frozen. Line the grill pan with foil to make washing-up easier.

5ml/1 tsp green peppercorns	15ml/1 tbsp lemon juice
10ml/1 dsp fresh chopped herbs	4 cod fillets
e.g. parsley, tarragon, dill, fennel	3ml/½ tsp paprika
30ml/2 tbsp olive oil	

1 Finely chop the peppercorns and mix along with the herbs in the oil and lemon juice.
2 Spread the mixture evenly over the cod fillets and sprinkle with the paprika.
3 Cook under a hot grill with the rack removed from the grillpan for approximately 10 minutes or until the fish is browning and just cooked. Do not turn over.

Grilled Fish with Tomato and Pesto

Serves 4

It is best to use homemade pesto sauce as the bought varieties usually contain cheese. Line the grillpan with foil to save on washing-up.

40ml/4 dsp olive oil	4 large tomatoes
40ml/4dsp lemon juice	10ml/1 dsp pesto sauce *(see*
1 clove garlic, pressed	*Chapter 8, page 202)*
4 pieces of fish	black pepper

1 Mix the oil, lemon juice and garlic. Pour over the fish and allow to marinade for at least 10 minutes.
2 Skin and finely dice the tomatoes, and mix with the pesto sauce and the pepper.
3 Cook the fish under a hot grill with the rack removed from the grill pan for approximately 10 minutes or until the fish is just cooked. Baste with the marinade during cooking.
4 Serve with the tomato and pesto mixture spread over the top of the fish.

Fried Fish

Serves 4

The corn flour gives the fish a lovely golden colour but you can use soya or rice flour if you cannot tolerate corn.

40ml/4 dsp corn flour	4 pieces filleted fish
black pepper	30ml/2 tbsp olive oil

1 Mix the corn flour and pepper on a plate.
2 Wash the fish, dry lightly with kitchen roll then dip into the corn flour until the fish is well coated on both sides.
3 Fry the fish in the olive oil until it is golden brown on both sides and cooked through.

Fish Parcels

Serves 4

Serve on rice, millet or quinoa accompanied by salad or cooked vegetables.

4 pieces fish (preferably thick)	1 large tomato
1 leek *or* 4 spring onions (scallions)	5ml/1 tsp grated orange rind
	juice of 1 orange
1 stick (stalk) celery	10ml/1 dsp lemon juice
1 carrot	5ml/1 tsp grated ginger
1 small courgette (zucchini)	black pepper
15ml/1 tbsp chopped parsley	

1 Place each piece of fish on a piece of foil approximately 25-cm/10-inch square.
2 Slice the leek or spring onions (scallions) into ½-cm/⅛-inch pieces.
3 Cut the celery and carrot into very fine matchstick pieces.
4 Thinly slice the courgette (zucchini).
5 Sprinkle the vegetables on top of the fish, along with the parsley.
6 Skin and finely dice the tomato and mix with the remaining ingredients. Pour over the fish and vegetables.
7 Lift the corners of the foil and twist to form parcels.
8 Place on a baking tray and bake at 400°F/200°C/Gas Mark 6 for approximately 15–20 minutes or until the fish is just cooked.

Fish Pie

If your diet allows, add a knob of butter to the mashed potatoes. If you cannot tolerate potatoes, try topping the fish pie with a mixture of mashed parsnip and cooked millet. Prawns do contain salt unless freshly cooked and shelled, but another fish or vegetable could be used instead.

900g/2 lb/6½ cups potatoes	WHITE SAUCE:
black pepper	30ml/2 level tbsp corn flour
455g/1 lb/2¼ cups cod *or*	(cornstarch) *or* rice flour
haddock	3ml/½ tsp mustard
115g/4 oz/1 cup prawns	285ml/½ pt/1⅓ cups soya *or*
55g/2 oz/¼ cup fresh *or* frozen	almond milk
peas	140ml/¼ pt/⅔ cup potato
55g/2 oz/¼ cup sweetcorn	cooking water
kernels	2ml/¼ tsp nutmeg
olive oil	5ml/1 tsp lemon juice
	3ml/½ tsp grated lemon rind
	15ml/1 tbsp chopped parsley
	black pepper

1 Peel and chop the potatoes and boil in water until soft. Mash using a little of the cooking liquid or some soya milk to give a soft consistency, and season with black pepper. Save the remaining cooking liquid to use in the white sauce.
2 To make the white sauce, mix the corn flour (cornstarch) or rice flour and mustard with a little milk in a saucepan. Add the rest of the milk, 140ml/¼ pint/⅔ cup of the potato water and the remaining sauce ingredients. Bring to the boil, stirring constantly, then lower the heat and simmer for 2 minutes.
3 Cut the fish into small pieces and add to the sauce along with the prawns, peas and sweetcorn, and mix gently.
4 Place the fish mixture into a gratin dish and spread the mashed potato over the top.

5 Brush the surface with olive oil and bake near the top of the oven at 400°F/200°C/Gas Mark 6 for 30 minutes. If the surface is not brown enough, place under a hot grill for a few minutes.

Seafood Pasta

Serves 4

Follow the previous recipe, but instead of topping with mashed potatoes, mix the fish sauce with cooked pasta. Use 225g/8 oz/2½ cups pasta, made from rice, corn or buckwheat.

Fish with Red Onions and Green Peppers

Serves 4

Serve with baked potatoes and a salad. The fish pieces could be baked together in a large gratin dish, but allow an extra 5 minutes cooking time.

4 red onions	4 thick pieces of fish (e.g. cod, haddock)
2 green peppers	
45ml/3 tbsp olive oil	30ml/2 tbsp lemon juice
	black pepper

1 Slice the onions into rings and the green peppers into strips.
2 Sweat the onions and peppers in 15ml/1 tbsp olive oil until they begin to soften and brown. This will take approximately 20 minutes. Stir frequently and do not be tempted to turn the heat up too high.
3 Divide the onion and pepper mixture between 4 small gratin dishes and place a piece of fish on top of the vegetables.
4 Mix the remaining 30ml/2 tbsp olive oil with the lemon juice and spread over the fish. Sprinkle with lots of black pepper.
5 Cover with foil and bake at 400°F/200°C/Gas Mark 6 for approximately 15 minutes or until the fish is just cooked.

Tuna and Lentil Bake

Serves 4

The surface could be sprinkled with grated cheese, if your diet allows.

170g/6 oz/1 cup red split lentils
1 large onion, diced
10ml/1 dsp olive oil
2 large eggs
140ml/¼ pint/⅔ cup soya *or* almond milk

200g/7 oz/1⅓ cups tuna in water
black pepper
30ml/2 tbsp chopped nuts

1 Wash the lentils and bring to the boil in a pan with 570ml/1 pint/2½ cups of water. Simmer for 20–25 minutes until the lentils are soft and most of the liquid has been absorbed.
2 Sweat the onion in the oil until it begins to soften.
3 Separate the eggs and beat the yolks and milk together. Whisk the egg whites until stiff.
4 Flake the tuna fish and include the juices from the tin.
5 Combine the lentils, onion, tuna, egg, milk and pepper. Fold in the egg whites using a metal spoon.
6 Pour the mixture into a shallow, greased ovenproof dish, sprinkle the surface with the nuts and bake at 350°F/180°C/Gas Mark 4 for 30 minutes or until the bake is set and brown.

Kedgeree

Serves 4

225g/8 oz/1 cup brown rice
2 large onions, diced
10ml/1 dsp olive oil
2 hardboiled eggs (optional)
225g/8 oz/1 cup fresh fish
55g/2 oz/½ cup prawns
15ml/1 tbsp fresh parsley

SAUCE:
30ml/2 tbsp fish cooking liquid
5ml/1 tsp curry powder
30ml/2 tbsp olive oil
80ml/4 tbsp mayonnaise *(see page 200) or* soya yogurt
15ml/1 tbsp lemon juice
3ml/½ tsp grated lemon rind

1 Cook the brown rice, sieve and keep warm.
2 Sweat the onions in the oil until they begin to soften and brown. Cut the eggs into rough dice.
3 In a pan poach the fish in 30ml/2 tbsp water until just cooked. Flake the fish and remove any skin or bones.
4 Mix the rice, fish, prawns, eggs, onions and parsley.
5 Make the sauce by blending 30ml/2 tbsp of the fish liquid with the curry powder and the oil. It is best to use a food processor, if available, in order to obtain a thick emulsion. Add the mayonnaise or yogurt and the lemon juice and rind.
6 Pour the sauce over the fish and rice and mix gently with a fork.

Fish Cakes

Serves 4

Substitute butter beans if you cannot eat eggs.

565g/1¼ lb/4 cups potatoes	30ml/2 tbsp chopped parsley
1 tin (400g/14oz/2 cups) tuna fish (in water)	20ml/2 dsp lemon juice
1 large onion	black pepper
2 hardboiled eggs	olive oil

1 Cook the potatoes in boiling water until soft. Mash using the drained water from the tuna to give a soft consistency.
2 Finely dice the onion and cook in 30ml/2 tbsp of water until soft. Sieve to remove the water.
3 Chop the hardboiled egg and stir into the potatoes along with the onion, tuna, parsley, lemon juice and black pepper.
4 Shape into 12 cakes and place on a well-greased baking tray. Brush the fish cakes with olive oil, and cook on the top shelf of a hot oven at 450°F/230°C/Gas Mark 8 for approximately 20 minutes or until brown.

Tuna, Butter Bean and Leek Savoury

Serves 4

455g/1 lb/4 cups leeks	2ml/¼ tsp ground nutmeg
1 large carrot	3ml/½ tsp grated lemon rind
140ml/¼ pint/⅔ cup water	10ml/1 dsp fresh parsley
200g/7 oz/1⅓ cups tinned tuna in water	black pepper
285ml/½ pint/1⅓ cups soya *or* almond milk	225g/8 oz/1 cup cooked butter beans
30ml/2 level tbsp corn flour (cornstarch)	15ml/1 tbsp chopped nuts

1 Slice the leeks and cut the carrot into matchstick pieces. Cook in 140ml/¼ pint/⅔ cup of water, sieve and save the cooking liquid.
2 Drain and flake the tuna fish, saving the juices from the tin.
3 Make the milk up to 425ml/¾ pint/2 cups with the tuna and vegetable liquids. Add a little water if necessary.
4 Mix the milk and corn flour (cornstarch) together in a pan until smooth. Bring to the boil, stirring constantly, and simmer for 2 minutes.
5 Mix all the ingredients except the nuts into the sauce, taking care when mixing the butter beans so that they do not break up.
6 Place the mixture into 1 large or 4 small gratin dishes. Sprinkle the surface with nuts and serve.

Quick Fish Casserole

Serves 4

Serve with rice, millet or quinoa and salad or vegetables.

1 carrot	black pepper
½ onion	10ml/1 dsp corn flour
10ml/1 dsp olive oil	(cornstarch)
4 portions fish (e.g. cod,	140ml/¼ pint/⅔ cup soya *or*
haddock, hake)	almond milk
140ml/¼ pint/⅔ cup water	80ml/4 tbsp frozen peas
1 bay leaf	

1 Grate the carrot and onion and sweat in the olive oil for 3 minutes.
2 Add the fish and turn to coat with the vegetables and oil. Add the water, the bay leaf and some black pepper. Cover the pan and cook gently until the fish is almost cooked, approximately 10 minutes.
3 Mix the corn flour (cornstarch) and milk to a smooth paste and add to the pan, mixing with the juices and vegetables. Bring to the boil, add the frozen peas, cover and cook gently for another 5 minutes.

Majorcan Fish Casserole

Serves 4

680g/1½ lb/5 cups potatoes (even sized)	1 tin (400g/15 oz/2 cups) chopped tomatoes in tomato juice
1 large onion	2ml/¼ tsp dried thyme
10ml/1 dsp olive oil	2ml/¼ tsp dried marjoram
1 courgette (zucchini)	3ml/½ tsp fennel seeds
225g/½ lb/4 cups spinach	black pepper
30ml/2 tbsp pine nuts	4 pieces cod *or* hake
30ml/2 tbsp raisins (optional)	olive oil for brushing the surface

1 Boil the potatoes whole in their skins for approximately 10–15 minutes, depending on the size of the potatoes. They should be slightly undercooked at this stage. Allow to cool.

2 Dice the onion and sweat in the olive oil until it begins to soften and brown. Dice the courgette (zucchini), add to the pan and sweat the vegetables for a few more minutes.

3 Chop the spinach and add to the onion and courgette (zucchini) along with the pine nuts, raisins, tomatoes, herbs and pepper. Bring to the boil and simmer for 5 minutes.

4 Place the mixture into 1 large or 4 small gratin dishes. Lay the fish pieces on top.

5 Skin the potatoes then grate them using a food processor or hand grater. Pile the grated potatoes on top of the fish, pressing down a little but leaving the surface quite rough.

6 Brush the surface with olive oil and bake at the top of the oven for approximately 15 minutes for the small dishes and 20 minutes for the larger at 400°F/200°C/Gas Mark 6. Place under a hot grill for 2 minutes if the potatoes have not browned sufficiently in the oven.

SaucesandDressingsSaucesand

SaucesandDressings

French Dressing

If your diet allows, 5ml/1 tsp of honey makes this dressing taste less sharp. If you do not like the taste of olive oil, use half sunflower oil, but gradually keep reducing the amount as you become accustomed to the taste of olive oil. If you cannot tolerate citrus fruits but can tolerate cider vinegar, use one-third vinegar and two-thirds olive oil.

juice of 1 orange
juice of 1 lemon
olive oil
10ml/1 dsp mustard
3ml/½ tsp lemon rind
black pepper
3ml/½ tsp orange rind

Choose 4 dried herbs from the
following:
3ml/½ tsp parsley
3ml/½ tsp dill seeds
3ml/½ tsp celery seeds
3ml/½ tsp mint
3ml/½ tsp chives

3ml/½ tsp fennel seeds
3ml/½ tsp tarragon

If substituting fresh herbs, use
5ml/1 tsp of each

Other flavourings which could
be added include:
3ml/½ tsp paprika
5ml/1 tsp tahini
5ml/1 tsp grated raw onion
5ml/1 tsp tomato purée
3ml/½ tsp grated ginger
1 clove garlic, pressed

1 Place the orange and lemon juice in a screw-topped jar and add an equal amount of olive oil.
2 Add the remaining ingredients and shake well.
3 Store in the fridge ready for use.

Tofu Mayonnaise

Flavour with garlic, curry powder, tomato purée, spring onion (scallion) or herbs, if desired.

1 packet (290g/10 oz/1 cup) silken tofu
15ml/1 tbsp lemon juice
5ml/1 tsp mustard

black pepper
170ml/6 fl oz/¾ cup oil (use a mixture of olive oil and sunflower)

1 Process the tofu, lemon juice, mustard and pepper in a food processor.
2 Slowly add the oils through the funnel of the food processor with the machine on full power.
3 Store the mayonnaise in a covered container in the fridge for up to 3 days.

Mayonnaise

The amount of oil needed varies according to the size of the eggs. I never measure the oil but just pour it from the bottle until the mayonnaise is the right thickness. Olive oil can be used on its own, but this produces quite a strong-flavoured mayonnaise.

Vary the mayonnaise by adding flavourings such as herbs, garlic, curry powder, tomato purée or spring onions (scallions).

15ml/1 tbsp lemon juice	black pepper
10ml/1 dsp mustard	approximately 170ml/6 fl oz/
2 egg yolks + 30ml/2 tbsp water	¾ cup oil (use a mixture of olive
or 1 whole egg	and sunflower)

1 Process all the ingredients except the oil in a food processor until well mixed.
2 Leave the food processor running on high power and *very* slowly add the oil a few drops at a time until it starts to emulsify. Then add the rest of the oil slowly until the desired thickness of mayonnaise is obtained.
3 Store in the fridge and use as required.

Thousand Island Mayonnaise

Add the following ingredients to the previous recipe for Mayonnaise and mix:

10ml/1 dsp finely chopped parsley	30ml/2 tbsp chopped green olives
10ml/1 dsp finely chopped onions *or* chives	30ml/2 tbsp finely chopped green pepper
10ml/1 dsp tomato purée	

White Sauce

30ml/2 level tbsp corn flour (cornstarch) or rice flour	3ml/½ tsp lemon rind
5ml/1 level tsp mustard	2ml/¼ tsp nutmeg
425ml/¾ pt/2 cups soya or almond milk	1 bay leaf
	black pepper

1 In a saucepan, mix the corn flour (cornstarch) or rice flour, mustard and a little milk together until smooth.
2 Add the remaining milk along with the lemon rind, nutmeg, bay leaf and black pepper.
3 Bring to the boil, stirring constantly. Simmer for 2 minutes.
4 Remove the bay leaf.

Parsley Sauce

Add 30ml/2 tbsp of finely chopped parsley to the previous recipe for White Sauce.

Onion Sauce

Boil a finely diced onion in 140ml/¼ pint/⅔ cup of water until soft. Drain, keep the liquid and use this instead of some of the milk in the recipe for White Sauce (see above). Add the onions to the cooked sauce along with lots of black pepper and the other ingredients.

Mushroom Sauce

Add 115g/4 oz/1 cup mushrooms, sliced and sautéed, to the White Sauce (see above).

Velouté Sauce

Use a good quality stock instead of half of the milk in the recipe for White Sauce *(see page 201).*

Pesto Sauce

55g/2 oz/2 cups fresh basil leaves	1 clove garlic
30g/1 oz/⅓ cup pine nuts	black pepper
	60ml/2 fl oz/¼ cup olive oil

1 Using a pestle and mortar or food processor, blend the basil, pine nuts, garlic and black pepper thoroughly, then gradually work in the olive oil to give a smooth mixture.
2 Store in the fridge.

Herb and Walnut Sauce

Substitute walnuts for the pine nuts in the previous recipe for Pesto Sauce, and a selection of herbs such as parsley, mint, chives, tarragon, coriander and dill instead of the basil leaves.

Serve 5ml/1 tsp mixed into a bowl of freshly boiled rice for a delicious snack. Pesto Sauce and Herb and Walnut Sauce can also be used to add flavour to risottos, soups and casseroles.

Ratatouille Sauce

Serve as a sauce or vegetable accompaniment.

½ aubergine (eggplant)	1 large tin (400g/15 oz/2 cups)
½ green pepper	chopped tomatoes in tomato
½ red pepper	juice
2 courgettes (zucchini)	285ml/½ pint/1⅓ cups water
1 large onion	3ml/½ tsp dried basil
	3ml/½ tsp dried oregano
	black pepper

1 Dice the aubergine (eggplant) and peppers and slice the courgettes (zucchini) and onion.
2 Place all the ingredients into a saucepan and bring to the boil.
3 Cover the pan and simmer for 40 minutes. Season with black pepper and serve.

Fresh Tomato Sauce

A large tin (400g/15 oz/2 cups) of chopped tomatoes could be substituted for the fresh ones.

½ small onion	30ml/2 tbsp chopped fresh
1 clove garlic	herbs e.g. parsley, chives, basil,
10ml/1 dsp olive oil	coriander, marjoram *or* 5ml/1
455g/1 lb/2½ cups fresh	tsp dried herbs, e.g. basil,
tomatoes	oregano
	3ml/½ tsp paprika
	black pepper

1 Finely dice the onion and press the garlic clove. Place the oil in a saucepan and sweat the garlic and onion for a few minutes until soft and beginning to brown.
2 Skin and chop the tomatoes and add to the pan.
3 Add the remaining ingredients and cook until the tomatoes have just melted, no more than 5 minutes.
4 Serve immediately with nut roasts, vegetables, rice etc.

Vegetable Purée Sauce

Serve with nut roasts, rice, fish or chicken. Fresh herbs could be added if desired, such as parsley, chives, basil, coriander, marjoram.

1 medium onion	285ml/½ pint/1⅓ cups water
4 large carrots	5ml/1 tsp lemon juice
2 large tomatoes	black pepper

1 Dice the onion and slice the carrots. Skin the tomatoes.
2 Cook the onion and carrot in the water until they are just soft, then allow to cool slightly.
3 Process the carrot, onion and water in a food processor until smooth. Add the tomatoes, lemon juice and pepper and process again.
4 Heat through but do not cook further.

Dahl

Use as a sauce for vegetarian roasts, or on its own with brown rice or Spicy Baked Chicken *(see Chapter 6, page 170)*. If your diet allows, 30ml/2 tbsp of yogurt can be added just before serving.

A variation on the above can be made by substituting whole green lentils for the red lentils and adding a finely diced onion. This dish is ideal to serve along with a meat dish and a vegetarian dish as part of an Indian-style meal.

200g/7 oz/1 cup red split lentils	2ml/¼ tsp cayenne pepper
1 clove garlic	3ml/½ tsp garam masala
3ml/½ tsp ground coriander	5ml/1 tsp grated ginger *or*
3ml/½ tsp turmeric	3ml/½ tsp ground ginger
5ml/1 tsp cumin seeds	1 litre/35 fl oz/4½ cups water

1 Wash the lentils, press the garlic clove and place all the ingredients in a saucepan. Bring to the boil.
2 Simmer gently, stirring occasionally, for 1½ hours.

Curry Sauce

Serve as a sauce to add flavour to rice, meat or vegetables. A vegetable curry can be made by adding 455g/1 lb/3–4 cups of chopped mixed vegetables and cooking in the sauce until tender. Alternatively, make an egg curry by hardboiling one egg per person and serving the egg halved, on top of rice, with the sauce poured over.

1 large onion	30g/1 oz/⅙ cup creamed
1 large baking apple	coconut
10ml/1 dsp olive oil	30ml/2 tbsp raisins (optional)
5ml/1 tsp curry powder	15ml/1 tbsp tomato purée
850ml/1½ pints/3¾ cups water	(optional)
55g/2 oz/⅓ cup red split lentils	

1 Dice the onion and grate the baking apple. Sweat the onion in the oil until it begins to soften and brown.
2 Add the grated apple and the curry powder and sweat for a few more minutes.
3 Add the remaining ingredients, bring to the boil and simmer, covered, for at least 1 hour until the lentils and apples have become part of a thick sauce. Stir occasionally during cooking and add a little more water if the sauce is too dry.

Chickpea and Avocado Sauce

Use as a sauce with rice, nut roasts, vegetables etc. or as a dip with vegetable crudités. Add more water if a softer sauce is required.

1 medium avocado	15ml/1 tbsp tahini
15ml/1 tbsp lemon juice	115g/4 oz/⅔ cup cooked
45ml/3 tbsp water	chickpeas
15ml/1 tbsp olive oil	

1 Process the avocado with the lemon juice, water and olive oil in a food processor.
2 Add the tahini and chickpeas and process until a smooth sauce is obtained.

Fennel and Cashew Nut Sauce

Serve with rice, millet, quinoa or pasta.

225g/8 oz/2 cups leeks	3ml/½ tsp grated ginger
225g/8 oz/2 cups fennel	black pepper
140ml/5 fl oz/⅔ cup water *or*	30ml/1 oz/¼ cup cashew nuts
stock	140ml/5 fl oz/⅔ cup soya *or*
3ml/½ tsp fennel seeds	almond milk

1 Slice the leeks, using mainly the white stems, and dice the fennel.
2 Bring to the boil in the water or stock, add the fennel seeds, the ginger and the pepper and simmer for 10 minutes.
3 In a food processor, process the cashew nuts until fine, then add the leek and fennel mixture and process again until the sauce is smooth and creamy.
4 Return to the pan along with the milk. Bring the sauce to the boil and serve.

Pea and Caraway Sauce

170g/6 oz/¾ cup dried | black pepper
marrowfat peas | 5ml/1 tsp caraway seeds
200ml/7 fl oz/¾ cup water |

1 Soak the peas overnight in lots of water. Rinse the peas, cover with boiling water, bring to the boil and cook until soft (this will only take approximately 10 minutes in a pressure cooker).
2 Drain off the excess liquid. Using this liquid and some extra water if necessary, measure out 200ml/7 fl oz/¾ cup and add this to the peas along with the pepper and caraway seeds.
3 Bring to the boil and simmer until the peas fall to form a sauce. Add a little more water if needed.

BakingWithoutBakingWithoutBaking

Because the baked goods in this section contain very little fat and no sugar, they will not keep for long. Store in the fridge and eat within three days. They may be cut into slices, or packed in small portions and stored in the freezer to be used as needed. If you cannot tolerate eggs, you will find a variety of egg replacers available in health-food shops, or make your own by following the recipe in the Introduction *(see page 42)*. Egg replacers will help to bind ingredients together but do not help mixtures to rise as do ordinary eggs. It may be necessary to add an extra 3ml/½ tsp baking powder in cakes and breads where a light texture is desired.

Potassium baking powder is also available in health-food shops, and should be used in place of ordinary baking powder in these recipes to avoid the use of excess sodium. If you cannot find either potassium baking powder or egg replacer in your local health-food shop then do ask as these are available from the wholesalers but may not have been requested before.

I have tried to use the more readily available flours, but others could be substituted. The range is continually increasing. Do experiment with other flours if you cannot use the ones suggested. Also try using alternative flours instead of wheat flour in some of your favourite recipes. For 170g/6 oz/1¼ cups of wheat flour, substitute 115g/4 oz/⅔ cup corn flour (cornstarch), 85g/3 oz/½ cup potato flour, 140g/5 oz/¾ cup rice flour or 85g/3 oz/1 cup soya flour.

It is difficult to make cakes without some form of sweetening, and so dried fruit has been used in quite a few of these recipes. I find that many individuals with *Candida albicans* can tolerate dried fruit if used sparingly, but some who have an intolerance or allergy to yeast will not be able to use any. These individuals could try using crystallized ginger and pineapple or dried apple to obtain some sweetness. Although the ginger and pineapple contain some sugar, they do not contain yeast, and it is probably better to use these than to abandon *Cooking Without* and end up eating a bar of chocolate in desperation for something sweet.

If possible, use scales to measure the ingredients for the following recipes as cup measurements may not be accurate enough to obtain good results. Similarly, it is best to use measuring spoons rather than the spoons in the cutlery drawer as these do vary a lot in size.

Fruit and Nut Slices

If you do not have a food processor, grate the carrot and apple finely and chop the nuts, then mix all the ingredients together. This produces a slice which is more chunky and chewy. These slices benefit from the rice being well cooked and are ideal to make with an overcooked batch. Cooked millet or quinoa can be used instead of rice. A baking or an eating apple can be used.

1 large carrot	2 eggs *or* egg replacer
1 large apple	115g/4 oz/⅔ cup rice flour
90ml/3 fl oz/⅓ cup water	55g/2 oz/½ cup raisins
3ml/½ tsp cinnamon	(optional)
3ml/½ tsp nutmeg	55g/2 oz/½ cup hazelnuts
225g/8 oz/1⅓ cups well-cooked brown rice	sesame *or* sunflower seeds to decorate

1 Line a shallow tin (approximately 30cm by 23cm or 12in by 9in) with greaseproof paper or foil and oil the surface.
2 Roughly chop the carrot and apple and place in a food processor with the water, spices, cooked rice and eggs. Process until quite smooth.
3 Add the rice flour and process to combine.
4 Add the fruit and nuts and process for approximately 10 seconds until the fruit and nuts are chopped a little but still in pieces.
5 Place the mixture into the prepared tin and smooth the surface. Mark into 16 sections and sprinkle the surface with sunflower or sesame seeds.
6 Bake at 400°F/200°C/Gas Mark 6 for 20 minutes.
7 Cool in the tin, then turn the slices over and peel off the paper or foil.
8 Store in an airtight container in the fridge and use within 3 days. Alternatively, pack in handy-sized portions and freeze ready for snacks to take to work or on outings.

Parsnip, Banana and Apricot Slices

Use the previous recipe but substitute the carrot with a parsnip, the raisins with chopped dried apricots and add 55g/2 oz/⅓ cup of banana to the mixture before processing.

Carob Slices

Carob slices, the Fruit and Nut and Slices (see page 213) and the Savoury Slices (see page 215) are all based on the same recipe which was invented by a patient of mine whose young children were on this dietary regime. She wanted them to be able to take something to school for break time which seemed an acceptable snack food. I make batches twice weekly and keep them in the fridge. There is then always something to take to work or to nibble whenever a snack is needed.

1 large carrot	55g/2 oz/½ cup carob flour
1 large apple	55g/2 oz/⅓ cup rice flour
90ml/3 fl oz/⅓ cup water	30g/1 oz/½ cup desiccated
225g/8 oz/1⅓ cups well-cooked	coconut
brown rice	55g/2 oz/½ cup raisins (optional)
2 eggs or egg replacer	55g/2 oz/½ cup hazelnuts
3ml/½ tsp mixed spice	sunflower seeds, to decorate

1 Line a shallow tin (approximately 30cm by 23cm or 12in by 9in) with greaseproof paper or foil and oil the surface.
2 Roughly chop the carrot and apple and place in a food processor along with the water, cooked rice, eggs and mixed spice. Process until well mixed and fairly smooth. Add the carob flour and rice flour and process to combine.
3 Add the coconut, raisins and hazelnuts and process for 10 seconds until the nuts and fruit are chopped a little but still in pieces.
4 Place the mixture in the prepared tin and smooth the surface. Mark into 16 sections and sprinkle the surface with sunflower seeds.
5 Bake at 400°F/200°C/Gas Mark 6 for 20 minutes.

6 Allow to cool in the tin, turn the slices over and peel off the paper or foil. Store in an airtight container in the fridge and use within 3 days or pack in small portions in the freezer.

Savoury Slices

If the sun-dried tomatoes are not in olive oil, soak first in a little water to soften. Use a baking or an eating apple.

1 large carrot	115g/4 oz/⅔ cup rice flour
1 large apple	30g/1 oz/¼ cup sunflower *or*
90ml/3 fl oz/⅓ cup water	pumpkin seeds
5ml/1 tsp fennel seeds	55g/2 oz/¼ cup sweetcorn
3ml/½ tsp dried tarragon	kernels *or* frozen peas
2ml/¼ tsp chilli powder	4 sun-dried tomatoes
225g/8 oz/1⅓ cups well-cooked	8 olives, quartered
brown rice	sesame *or* poppy seeds to garnish
2 eggs *or* egg replacer	black pepper

1 Line a shallow tin (approximately 30cm by 23cm or 12in by 9in) with foil or greaseproof paper. Oil the surface.
2 Roughly chop the carrot and apple and place in a food processor with the water, herbs and spices, the cooked brown rice and the eggs. Process until well mixed and fairly smooth. Add the rice flour and process to combine.
3 Tip the mixture out into a bowl and mix in the sunflower or pumpkin seeds, the sweetcorn, the finely chopped sun-dried tomatoes and the olives.
4 Spread into the prepared tin and smooth the surface. Mark into 16 sections and sprinkle the surface with sesame or poppy seeds and lots of freshly ground black pepper.
5 Bake at 400°F/200°C/Gas Mark 6 for 20 minutes.
6 Allow to cool in the tin then turn the slices over and peel off the paper or foil. Store in an airtight container in the fridge and eat within 3 days or freeze and use as needed.

Apple, Date and Nut Muffins

These muffins are delicious and a real treat for anyone who misses cakes. Do not, however, eat too many of them as they are high in fruit sugar. Individuals with *Candida* problems may need to resist these in the early stages of treatment.

The mixture can be cooked as a loaf by placing in a greased and lined loaf tin and baking for 1¼ hours at 350°F/180°C/Gas Mark 4. Remove from the tin, peel off the lining paper and cool on a wire tray.

225g/8 oz/2 cups cooking apples, weighed after peeling	2ml/¼ tsp nutmeg
55g/2 oz/½ cup sultanas	225g/8 oz/1⅓ cups rice flour
55g/2 oz/½ cup chopped dates	20ml/2 level dsp baking powder
55g/2 oz/½ cup chopped walnuts	15ml/1 tbsp sunflower oil
2ml/½ tsp cinnamon	240ml/8 fl oz/1 cup water
	1 egg *or* egg replacer

1 Cut the apple into 2-cm/½-inch dice and place in a bowl with the fruit and nuts.
2 Place the remaining ingredients in a food processor and process until smooth. If you do not have a food processor, beat together in a bowl.
3 Combine the two sets of ingredients.
4 Pile into 12 greased bun or muffin tins. The mixture will be piled up high if using bun tins but this will be fine.
5 Bake for approximately 20 minutes at 400°F/200°C/Gas Mark 6.
6 Remove from the tins and place on a wire tray to cool. Store in the fridge and eat within 3 days. The muffins can be frozen if desired.

Banana, Date and Nut Loaf

Substitute 225g/8 oz/1¾ cups of chopped banana for the apple in the previous recipe.

Ginger and Orange Cake

If allowed, add crystallized ginger and candied peel instead of the sultanas for a really delicious but not too sinful cake. Individuals with *Candida albicans* may cope better with ginger than with dried fruit. If using an egg replacer, extra water may be needed to make the mixture into a soft consistency. Raw courgette (zucchini) can be used instead of the banana in this recipe.

1 egg *or* an egg replacer
115g/4 oz/⅔ cup potato flour
55g/2 oz/⅓ cup rice flour
55g/2 oz/⅔ cup ground almonds
15ml/1 tbsp sunflower oil
55g/2 oz/⅓ cup banana
juice of 1 orange made up to
170ml/6 fl oz/¾ cup with water

5ml/1 tsp grated orange rind
5ml/1 tsp ground ginger
20ml/2 level dsp baking powder
85g/3 oz/¾ cup sultanas
(optional)

1 If a food processor is available, place all the ingredients except the sultanas into the goblet and process until smooth and well mixed. Alternatively, beat the egg in a bowl and add the remaining ingredients, beating well with a wooden spoon.
2 Add and mix in the sultanas.
3 Place the mixture in a small greased loaf tin and bake in the centre of the oven at 400°F/200°C/Gas Mark 6 for approximately 30 minutes or until golden brown and firm to the touch.
4 Turn out of the tin and cool on a wire tray. Keep in a covered container in the fridge and eat within 3 days or freeze in slices.

Carrot and Coconut Cake

If using an egg replacer, extra water may be needed to make the mixture into a soft consistency. Use grated courgette (zucchini) instead of the carrot if desired.

1 egg *or* an egg replacer	170ml/6 fl oz/¾ cup warm water
170g/6 oz/1 cup finely grated carrot	140g/5 oz/¾ cup brown rice flour
55g/2 oz/⅔ cup desiccated coconut	20ml/2 level dsp baking powder
3ml/½ tsp nutmeg	85g/3 oz/¾ cup sultanas (optional)
3ml/½ tsp cinnamon	1 egg *or* an egg replacer
15ml/1 tbsp sunflower oil	

1 If a processor is available, blend all the ingredients except the sultanas until smooth and well mixed. Alternatively, beat the egg in a bowl, add the other ingredients and beat well with a wooden spoon. Add and mix in the sultanas.

2 Place the mixture in a small greased loaf tin and bake in the centre of the oven at 400°F/200°C/Gas Mark 6 for approximately 40 minutes or until firm to the touch and golden brown.

3 Turn out of the tin and cool on a wire tray. Keep in a covered container in the fridge and eat within 3 days, or freeze in slices.

Potato Flour Bread

If an egg replacer is used, extra water may be needed to make the mixture into a soft consistency.

1 egg *or* an egg replacer	170ml/6 fl oz/¾ cup warm water
115g/4 oz/⅔ cup potato flour	15ml/1 tbsp sunflower oil
55g/2 oz/⅓ cup rice flour	20ml/2 level dsp baking powder
55g/2 oz/⅔ cup soya flour	

1 If a food processor is available, place all the ingredients into the goblet and process until smooth and well mixed. Alternatively, beat the egg in a bowl and add the remaining ingredients, beating well with a wooden spoon.
2 Place in a small greased loaf tin and bake at 400°F/200°C/Gas Mark 6 for 30–35 minutes or until firm to the touch and golden brown.
3 Remove from the tin and cool on a wire tray. Store in an airtight container in the fridge and eat within 3 days.

Cornbread

If an egg replacer is used, extra water may be needed to make the mixture into a soft consistency.

1 egg *or* an egg replacer	55g/2 oz/⅓ cup potato flour
½ small baking apple	115ml/4 fl oz/½ cup warm water
115g/4 oz/⅔ cup medium maize	15ml/1 tbsp sunflower oil
meal *or* polenta flour	20ml/2 level dsp baking powder

1 Mix all the ingredients together in a food processor or, if mixing by hand, beat the egg and grate the apple, then beat in the remaining ingredients with a wooden spoon.
2 Place in a small greased loaf tin and bake at 400°F/200°C/Gas Mark 6 for 35 minutes.
3 Remove from the tin, cool on a wire tray and store in the fridge in an airtight container. Eat within 3 days.

Onion and Herb Loaf

5ml/1 level tsp mustard
310ml/11 fl oz/1⅓ cups warm
water *or* 260ml/9 fl oz/1 cup
warm water plus 1 egg
115g/4 oz/⅔ cup rice flour
55g/2 oz/⅓ cup maize meal *or*
polenta flour
55g/2 oz/⅔ cup soya flour

5ml/1 tsp dried parsley
2ml/¼ tsp dried thyme
3 ml/½ tsp dried sage
20ml/2 level dsp baking powder
15ml/1 tbsp olive oil
2 spring onions (scallions) *or*
15ml/1 tbsp minced onion

1 If using a food processor, place all the ingredients in the goblet and process until smooth and well mixed. If mixing by hand, place the mustard in a bowl and beat with a little water until smooth. Add the remaining ingredients and beat well with a wooden spoon.

2 Place the mixture in a small greased loaf tin and bake in the centre of the oven at 400°F/200°C/Gas Mark 6 for approximately 40 minutes until the loaf is brown and firm to the touch.

3 Remove from the tin and cool on a wire tray. Store in the fridge in an airtight container and eat within 3 days.

Onion and Herb Focaccia Bread

In this recipe the previous bread ingredients are baked in a pizza-like base covered with herbs, garlic and olives.

1 small onion	Onion and Herb Loaf mixture
15ml/1 tbsp olive oil	*(see page 221)*
2 cloves garlic	30ml/2 tbsp fresh chopped
8 olives (optional)	herbs e.g. thyme, marjoram,
3 sun-dried tomatoes	parsley, rosemary, chives *or*
	5ml/1 tsp dried herbs

1 Cut the onion in half and then into paper-thin slices. Place in a bowl and mix to coat with the olive oil.
2 Cut the garlic into very thin slices and the olives in half.
3 Cut the sun-dried tomatoes into small pieces.
4 Grease two baking trays. Make the Onion and Herb Loaf mixture and spread into two 23-cm/9-inch rounds on the trays.
5 Spread the onion, garlic, olives, tomatoes and herbs over the surface and bake near the top of the oven at 400°F/200°C/Gas Mark 6 for 25–30 minutes until the bread is quite brown and crisp. Serve whilst still hot with salads or soup.

Spiced Carrot Bread

If using an egg replacer, extra water may be needed to make the mixture into a soft consistency. Courgettes (zucchini) could be used to replace the carrot in this recipe.

1 egg *or* egg replacer	3ml/½ tsp nutmeg
140g/5oz/¾ cup rice flour *or* millet flour	3ml/½ tsp cinnamon
170g/6 oz/1 cup finely grated carrot	90ml/3 fl oz/⅓ cup warm water
	20ml/2 level dsp baking powder
	15ml/1 tbsp sunflower oil

1 If a food processor is available, place all the ingredients into the goblet and process until they are well mixed and smooth. Alternatively, beat the egg in a bowl and add the remaining ingredients, beating well with a wooden spoon.
2 Place the mixture in a small greased loaf tin and bake for approximately 35–40 minutes at 400°F/200°C/Gas Mark 6, or until firm to the touch and beginning to brown.
3 Turn out onto a wire tray to cool. Store in an airtight container in the fridge and eat within 3 days.

Almond and Soya Biscuits

60ml/4 level tbsp carrot purée
45g/1½ oz/½ cup soya flour
115g/4 oz/1⅓ cups ground
almonds

¼ tsp natural almond essence
sunflower seeds to decorate

1 Cook a medium-sized carrot until tender. Purée in the food processor, then measure out 60ml/4 tbsp.
2 Mix the carrot purée, soya flour, ground almonds and almond
   essence in the food processor until you have a thick, sticky mixture.
3 Press together any loose pieces and roll out by hand into a sausage
   shape, approximately 3 cm/1 inch in diameter. Use a little soya
   flour if necessary to stop the mixture sticking.
4 Cut into thin slices, approximately ½ cm/⅛ inch thick using a sharp
   knife. There should be approximately 30 slices.
5 Lay the biscuits on a greased baking sheet. Press a few sunflower
   seeds into the surface of each biscuit.
6 Bake at 350°F/180°C/Gas Mark 4 for 20 minutes until beginning to
   brown and crisp around the edges.
7 Cool on a wire tray, then store in an airtight container and eat
   within 3 days.

Chewy Fruit Bars

This recipe may not be suitable for those with severe *Candida* problems or an intolerance to yeast as the dried fruit cannot be substituted.

115g/4 oz/½ cup dried apricots	6 puffed rice cakes *or* 55g/
115ml/4 fl oz/½ cup orange	2 oz/2 cups puffed rice cereal
juice *or* water	115g/4 oz/1¼ cups ground
5ml/1 tsp grated orange rind	almonds
55g/2 oz/½ cup nuts e.g.	55g/2 oz/½ cup dried fruit e.g.
almonds, hazelnuts	raisins, apple, peach
55g/2 oz/⅔ cup desiccated	extra desiccated coconut
coconut	

1 Cut the apricots into small pieces and simmer in the orange juice and orange rind or water for approximately 5 minutes or until soft.
2 Chop the nuts into small pieces and toast in the oven or under the grill. Toast the desiccated coconut in the same way but be careful that it does not burn.
3 Break the puffed rice cakes into pieces. Place these or the puffed rice cereal in the food processor goblet. Add the coconut, the ground almonds, the apricot mixture and process until well mixed. You will need to stop the machine and scrape the mixture from the sides of the bowl once or twice as the mixture is quite sticky.
4 Turn the mixture out into a bowl and add the chopped toasted nuts and the chopped dried fruit. Mix by hand until the mixture forms a large ball.
5 Line a baking tray with foil or greaseproof paper and sprinkle with desiccated coconut. Spread the mixture out, levelling the surface, and sprinkle with more coconut. Press down well, cut into 12 or 16 pieces then leave to dry out, preferably overnight, before storing in an airtight container. Use within 1 week.

Nutty Carob Snacks

55g/2 oz/⅔ cup desiccated coconut	3 puffed rice cakes *or* 30g/ 1 oz/1 cup puffed rice cereal
55g/2 oz/½ cup carob flour	90ml/6 tbsp nut butter e.g.
115g/4 oz/1⅓ cups ground almonds	almond, cashew etc. approximately 60ml/4 tbsp water

1 Place all the ingredients except the water into a food processor and mix well. Add sufficient water for the mixture to bind together when pressed.
2 Roll the mixture into walnut-sized balls and place on a tray. Leave to dry out overnight then store in an airtight container. Use within 1 week.

Popcorn

80ml/3 rounded tbsp poporn

Method 1

Place the popcorn in a large bowl and cover with a large plate. Microwave on the highest setting for approximately 5 minutes until the popcorn has stopped popping.

Method 2

Heat 10ml/1 dsp of olive oil in a heavy-bottomed pan until hot. Add the corn, cover the pan with a lid and keep on a high heat until the corn has finished popping. Shake the pan regularly to prevent the corn sticking and burning.

Carob Birthday Cake

This cake contains rather too much oil to eat on a daily basis but enables you to celebrate special occasions without feeling the odd one out.

The above mixture can be made into 12 deep buns which will need cooking for approximately 20 minutes. The potato flour can be omitted and extra rice flour used if desired. An egg replacer does not substitute well in this recipe as it is difficult to make a light cake without eggs. If you do use one, add an extra 5ml/1 tsp baking powder.

55g/2 oz/⅓ cup banana, sliced	20ml/2 level dsp baking powder
2 eggs	115ml/4 oz/½ cup sunflower oil
55g/2 oz/½ cup carob flour	105ml/7 tbsp soya milk *or* water
45g/1½ oz/¼ cup potato flour	toasted nuts *or* desiccated
70g/2½ oz/½ cup rice flour	coconut, to decorate

1 In a food processor, mix all the ingredients until smooth. Alternatively, mash the banana well then add the beaten eggs and the remaining ingredients, beating well with a wooden spoon. Sieve the carob flour if it is lumpy.
2 Place in a greased, lined 18-cm/7-inch sandwich tin and bake in the middle of the oven at 330°F/170°C/Gas Mark 3 for 50–60 minutes. Do not undercook or the cake will tend to deflate on cooling.
3 Turn out onto a wire tray and cool.
4 When cool, cut the cake into 3 layers and sandwich together with carob cream made with 115ml/4 fl oz/½ cup of water instead of 140ml/5 fl oz/⅔ cup *(see Chapter 10, page 236)*. Top with carob cream and decorate with toasted nuts or desiccated coconut. Carob chocolate could be used to decorate the cake but check the list of ingredients first.

Christmas Cake

This cake contains too much oil and dried fruit to be eaten often but is delicious for special occasions. Salt-free butter can be used to replace the oil.

170g/6 oz/1⅙ cups dried dates
140ml/5 fl oz/⅔ cup water
115ml/4 fl oz/½ cup sunflower oil
30g/1 oz/⅓ cup ground almonds
5 ml/1 tsp mixed spice
3 eggs *or* egg replacer

55g/2 oz/⅓ cup rice flour
55g/2 oz/⅔ cup soya flour
55g/2 oz/⅓ cup corn flour (cornstarch)
455g/1 lb/3 cups mixed dried fruit e.g. raisins, currants, sultanas

1 Chop the dates into small pieces and place in a pan with the water. Bring to the boil and simmer over a low heat for approximately 10 minutes until the dates are soft. Cool.
2 Process or beat together the dates, oil, ground almonds, spice, eggs and flours until they are well blended.
3 Stir in the dried fruit and mix well by hand.
4 Place into a lined and greased 18-cm/6–8-inch cake tin and bake at 330°F/170°C/Gas Mark 3 for approximately 30 minutes, then lower the temperature to 290°F/145°C/Gas Mark 1 for a further 45 minutes.
5 Allow the cake to cool for 10 minutes in the tin, then turn out onto a wire tray. Remove the lining paper and allow to cool. Store in the fridge and eat within 2 weeks, or freeze in slices.

Almond Paste

55g/2 oz/½ cup dried dates
60ml/2 fl oz/¼ cup water

115g/4 oz/1⅓ cups ground almonds
¼ tsp natural almond essence

1 Finely chop the dates and simmer in the water on a low heat until soft.
2 Process the dates, almonds and essence until the mixture starts to bind together. Press together any loose pieces and roll the mixture into a ball by hand.
3 Roll out the almond paste in rice flour to fit the Christmas Cake. Decorate with nuts if desired.

Simnel Cake

Use half the almond paste, roll out into a circle and sandwich in the middle of the Christmas Cake mixture before cooking. Cook as above. When cool, use the remaining almond paste to decorate the top.

Mincemeat

225g/8 oz/1¼ cups dried apricots
565g/1¼ lb/5 cups cooking apples
juice of 1 large orange
grated rind of 1 orange
3ml/½ tsp ground ginger
3ml/½ tsp nutmeg
3ml/½ tsp cinnamon
340ml/12 fl oz/1½ cups water
455g/1 lb/3 cups mixed dried fruit e.g. raisins, currants, sultanas

1 Finely chop the dried apricots and grate the apples.
2 Put all the ingredients into a saucepan, bring to the boil and simmer gently for approximately 20 minutes, stirring occasionally to prevent sticking. Allow to cool.
3 Store in jars for no more than 3 weeks in the fridge and up to 6 months in the freezer.

Mince Pies

12 Pies

PASTRY INGREDIENTS:	90ml/6 tbsp water
55g/2 oz/⅔ cup ground almonds	60ml/4 tbsp sunflower oil
170g/6 oz/1 cup rice flour	60ml/4 level tbsp nut butter
3ml/½ tsp cinnamon	(almond, cashew *or* hazelnut)
2ml/¼ tsp ground cloves	

1 Place all the ingredients into the food processor and blend until well mixed. The mixture will still resemble breadcrumbs but will form into a pastry as you press it together by hand. If you do not have a food processor, mix the dry ingredients together, then the wet ingredients. Combine the two sets of ingredients with a fork, then press together by hand.

2 Divide the pastry in half and roll out each half sandwiched between clingfilm. This helps to prevent the pastry from breaking.

3 At this point you can either wrestle with the pastry to make small mince pies or give in to the fact that the pastry is quite brittle and make a large plate pie. You may still have to patch the pie but do not worry – it will taste fine.

4 Use the mincemeat (see page 230) to fill the pie or pies, cover with a pastry lid and press the pastry together at the edges.

5 Bake at 350°F/180°C/Gas Mark 4 for approximately 10–15 minutes for small pies and 20–25 minutes for the large pie until golden brown and crisp.

DessertsDessertsDessertsDesserts

DessertsDessertsDesserts Desserts

I have tried to include a good selection of desserts so that treats are available for weekends, for entertaining or for those evenings when you just feel like something special. It has been necessary, however, to include dried fruits, tropical fruits and acidic fruits in quite a few recipes. As these desserts should not be eaten too regularly, try to eat starters rather than puddings on most days, and save desserts for the occasional meal.

Individuals with severe *Candida* problems or a yeast intolerance should avoid the recipes containing dried fruit.

Apricot and Banana Cheesecake

Serves 4

BASE:	TOPPING:
45g/1½ oz/⅓ cup hazelnuts	55g/2 oz/¼ cup dried apricots
30g/1 oz/⅓ desiccated coconut	85g/3 oz/½ cup banana, chopped
1 rice cake *or* 80ml/4 tbsp puffed rice cereal	290g/10oz packet/1¼ cups firm silken tofu
	2ml/¼ tsp cinnamon
	2ml/¼ tsp grated lemon rind
	hazelnuts, to decorate

To make the base:

1 Toast the hazelnuts and coconut separately, either in the oven or under the grill, until golden brown. Allow to cool then rub the skins off the hazelnuts.

2 Place all the base ingredients into a food processor until the nuts are finely chopped and all the ingredients are mixed. Remove from the processor.

To make the topping:

1 Cut the apricots into small pieces and simmer in a small amount of water until soft. Sieve to remove the cooking liquid.

2 Process the apricots, banana, tofu, cinnamon and lemon rind until smooth.

To assemble:

1 Alternate two layers of both the base and topping ingredients (finishing with a layer of topping) either in a dish or, preferably, in four tall glasses or sundae dishes. Decorate with a few hazelnuts and serve.

Carob Cream

Serves 4

Serve in sundae glasses decorated with toasted split almonds, or as a topping for other desserts.

115g/4 oz/¾ cup cashew nuts	2 large bananas
140ml/5 fl oz/⅔ cup water *or*	toasted split almonds to
soya *or* rice milk	decorate
15ml/1 tbsp carob powder	

1 Place the cashew nuts in a food processor for 2 minutes or until finely ground.
2 Add the remaining ingredients and process until smooth and creamy.

Carob Cream Dessert

Serves 4

Follow the recipe for Apricot and Banana Cheesecake *(see page 235)* but use the ingredients for Carob Cream *(see above)* instead of the apricot and banana topping. Assemble as before.

Apple Crumble

Serves 4

Serve hot with Vanilla Custard *(see page 244)*, soya yogurt or Banana and Mango Ice Cream *(see page 251)*. If you prefer a sharper taste, substitute baking apples for two eating apples. Oat flakes could be used instead of the millet flakes if gluten is acceptable. Other fruit can be substituted for the apples, such as plums or cherries, but the fruit needs to be naturally sweet as no sugar is added.

4 eating apples	30g/1 oz/⅓ cup desiccated coconut
30ml/2 tbsp water	
85g/3 oz/1 cup millet flakes	3ml/½ tsp cinnamon
30g/1 oz/⅙ cup brown rice flour	20ml/2 dsp sunflower oil
55g/2 oz/⅔ cup ground almonds	30ml/2 tbsp sunflower seeds

1 Peel and core the apples and finely slice into an ovenproof dish. Pour the water over the apples.
2 To make the crumble, place the millet flakes, rice flour, ground almonds, coconut and cinnamon into a bowl and rub in the oil by hand. Spread the crumble over the fruit and sprinkle the sunflower seeds on top.
3 Bake for 20 minutes at 400°F/200°C/Gas Mark 6 until the topping is brown and the apples are tender.

Apple Pie

Serves 4

The pastry in this pie is really crisp and delicious but difficult to handle. I find it easier to make saucer pies rather than one big pie. Use baking apples if you prefer a sharper taste or a mixture of the two. Serve with Vanilla Custard *(see page 244)*, soya yogurt or Banana and Mango Ice Cream *(see page 251)*. Try pies made from other sweet fruits, such as plums, cherries and blackberries, or make open-topped small pies filled with fresh fruit, such as strawberries, peaches, raspberries, kiwi fruit, etc.

1 portion pastry *(see recipe for Mince Pies, page 231)*	3ml/½ tsp cinnamon
4 eating apples	2ml/¼ tsp ground cloves

1 Follow the instructions for making pastry from the Mince Pie recipe and use half the pastry to line a pie dish.
2 Peel and core the apples and finely slice into the pie. Sprinkle the apples with the spices. Cover the pie with the remaining pastry, wetting the edges to seal the pie.
3 Bake at 350°F/180°C/Gas Mark 4 for approximately 20–25 minutes or until the pastry is golden brown and crisp and the filling cooked.

Baked Apples

Serves 4

Serve hot with Vanilla Custard *(see page 244)*, soya yogurt or just as they are. The apples could be stuffed with dried fruit before baking, if this is tolerated.

4 eating apples	grated rind of ½ orange
90ml/3 fl oz/⅓ cup orange juice, apple juice *or* water	3ml/½ tsp grated ginger
	3ml/½ tsp mixed spice

1 Wash and core the apples. Place in a casserole dish that is not too large so that the apples are supported by the sides. Prick the skins with a knife to prevent them bursting.
2 Mix the fruit juice or water with the orange rind, the ginger and the mixed spice, and pour around the apples in the casserole dish.
3 Cover the apples and bake in the centre of the oven at 400°F/ 200°C/Gas Mark 6 for approximately 30 minutes until the apples are just soft but not mushy.

Rice Pudding

Serves 4

15ml/1 tbsp chopped dates (optional)
90ml/3 fl oz/⅓ cup water
570ml/1 pint/2½ cups soya *or* almond milk
115g/4 oz/1 cup brown rice flakes

3ml/½ tsp ground cinnamon
30g/1 oz/¼ cup sultanas (optional)
4 drops natural vanilla extract *or* 1 vanilla pod
grated nutmeg

1 Place the chopped dates in the water and simmer until they are soft and mushy. Mix in the milk a little at a time, beating the dates well so that they disintegrate, sweetening the milk.
2 Place the milk, rice flakes, cinnamon, sultanas and vanilla into a greased casserole dish. Sprinkle the surface liberally with grated nutmeg.
3 Bake at 400°F/200°C/Gas Mark 6 for approximately 1 hour, stirring occasionally.

Almond Fruit Bake

Serves 4

Ground rice is not the same as rice flour. It is more coarsely ground. In winter, when a good selection of fresh fruit is not available, try serving with a mixture of fresh and stewed fruit, such as prune and pear or apricot and apple.

30g/1 oz/⅙ cup ground rice	680g/1½ lb/3–4 cups mixed
570ml/1 pint/2½ cups soya *or* almond milk	fresh sweet fruit e.g. cherries, apples, pears, peaches, apricots,
85g/3 oz/1 cup ground almonds	plums
3ml/½ tsp natural vanilla extract	

1 Mix the ground rice with 60ml/2 fl oz/¼ cup of cold milk. Bring the remaining milk to the boil, then add the ground rice mixture, stirring all the time until it returns to the boil. Simmer, stirring constantly, for 2 minutes.
2 Add the ground almonds and vanilla extract and stir well.
3 Pour into a shallow greased gratin dish.
4 Remove the stones or cores from the fruit where necessary and slice the larger fruits. Arrange the fruit on top of the ground rice mixture in an attractive pattern, placing the cut sides downwards. Press the fruit down well.
5 Bake for approximately 30 minutes, or until the fruit is cooked, at 400°F/200°C/Gas Mark 6. Serve hot or cold.

Stuffed Peaches

Serves 4

This is a really easy but quite delicious dessert, especially if served with Mango and Banana Ice Cream *(see page 251)*.

Almond Paste *(see Chapter 9, page 229)*
4 large peaches

30ml/2 tbsp toasted slivered almonds

1 Make the Almond Paste as directed.
2 Halve and stone the peaches and place in a baking dish, cut side uppermost (cut a little slice off the rounded edge, if necessary, to help them remain stable).
3 Divide the Almond Paste into 8 pieces, roll into balls and place a ball in the centre of each peach half.
4 Bake, covered, for 10 minutes, then uncovered for a further 10 minutes at 400°F/200°C/Gas Mark 6. The peaches should be soft and the filling just starting to brown.
5 Sprinkle with toasted slivered almonds before serving either hot or cold.

Fried Bananas

Serves 4

This is a very simple and easy to prepare dessert whose taste belies its simple ingredients. Serve with Vanilla Custard *(see page 244)*, Banana and Mango Ice Cream *(see page 251)*, soya yogurt or just as they are. If your diet allows dairy produce, use low-salt butter to fry the bananas for added flavour.

4 bananas	3ml/½ tsp cinnamon
5ml/1 tsp sunflower oil	juice of 1 orange
3ml/½ tsp grated lemon rind	15ml/1 tbsp toasted slivered
3ml/½ tsp grated orange rind	almonds

1 Peel the bananas and fry quickly in the oil until beginning to brown and soften on the outside. This will take only 2–3 minutes.
2 Add the remaining ingredients, mix well and serve immediately.

Vanilla Custard

Serves 4

If you cannot tolerate eggs, use 60ml/4 level tbsp corn flour (cornstarch) instead of the 30ml/2 tbsp in the list of ingredients. A vanilla pod could be used instead of the vanilla extract. The dates can be omitted if dried fruit is not acceptable.

30ml/2 tbsp finely chopped dates (optional)	570ml/1 pint/2½ cups soya *or* almond milk
60ml/2 fl oz/¼ cup water	2 eggs, beaten
30ml/2 tbsp corn flour (cornstarch)	3ml/½ tsp natural vanilla extract

1 Place the dates in the water in a saucepan and simmer until they are soft. Mix the corn flour (cornstarch) and the milk and add to the dates a little at a time, beating well to enable the dates to disintegrate and sweeten the milk.
2 Add the eggs and vanilla extract.
3 Gradually bring the mixture to the boil, stirring constantly. Lower the heat and simmer for 1 minute. Do not boil rapidly or the eggs will curdle.

Sponge and Custard

Serve the Vanilla Custard with warm Carrot and Coconut Cake *(see Chapter 9, page 218)*, Apple, Date and Nut Muffins *(see Chapter 9, page 216)* or Ginger and Orange Cake *(see Chapter 9, page 217)*.

Prunes and Custard

Serve the Vanilla Custard with stewed prunes.

Banana Custard

Cut 4 bananas into slices and add to the Vanilla Custard when it has cooled a little. Serve warm or allow to cool before serving.

Black Forest Trifle

Crumble ⅓ of a carob birthday cake into a serving dish. Mix in two small tins of fruit in natural juice ie. strawberries, raspberries, blackberries. Pour over vanilla custard and allow to cool. Serve with soya cream, if acceptable.

Baked Egg Custard

Serves 4

The custard will continue cooking for a little while once out of the oven, so remove while still a little soft. Serve with stewed dried fruit, Fried Bananas *(see page 243)* or Fresh Fruit Salad *(see page 248)*. A vanilla pod could be used instead of the extract but will need soaking in the warm milk for 30 minutes to allow the flavour to be absorbed. Remove the pod before baking.

3 eggs, beaten	3ml/½ tsp natural vanilla extract
570ml/1 pint/2½ cups soya *or* almond milk	nutmeg

1 Grease an ovenproof dish and put in the beaten eggs.
2 Warm the milk in a saucepan, then pour over the eggs, stirring thoroughly.
3 Mix in the vanilla extract and sprinkle the surface with nutmeg.
4 Place the dish in a baking tray containing cold water. Then place the two dishes in the oven.
5 Bake at 325°F/170°C/Gas Mark 3 for approximately 30 minutes or until the mixture is just setting in the centre. Do not overcook or the mixture will boil and curdle.

Fruit Fool

Serves 4

Serve in sundae glasses either just as it is or decorated with chopped nuts.

115g/4 oz/¾ cup cashew nuts 140ml/5 fl oz/⅔ cup soya *or* almond milk	455g/1 lb/4 cups fresh *or* frozen sweet fruit e.g. apricots, peaches, cherries, strawberries, plums, apples

1 Place the cashew nuts in a food processor until finely ground.
2 Add the milk and process again until a smooth cream is obtained.
3 If using soft fresh fruit, such as peaches or strawberries, add these to the cashew cream and process again. If using harder fresh fruit, such as apples or plums, stew the fruit in a little water until soft and add to the cashew cream, reserving the cooking liquid unless needed to make the mixture soft. If using frozen fruit, defrost and add to the cashew cream, again reserving any juices unless needed.

Fruit Fool Ice Cream

Serves 4

Follow the previous recipe but use frozen fruit. Do not defrost but add to the cashew nut cream through the processor funnel while the machine is on high power. Process until smooth and serve immediately or return to the freezer.

Fresh Fruit Salad

Serves 4

To liven up a fresh fruit salad in winter, use a little frozen fruit, such as raspberries and blackberries, or an occasional tin of fruit in natural juice as a base.

You do not have to use all the fruits available for a fruit salad. Try just serving 2–3 fruits, such as:

- melon and strawberry
- melon, kiwi fruit and blackberry
- melon and black grape

- pear, sharon fruit and raspberries
- orange and date

285ml/10 fl oz/1⅓ cups fresh fruit juice e.g. apple, orange, pineapple	plums
	sharon fruit
	strawberries
680g/1½ lb/3–4 cups fresh fruit selected from the following:	banana
	grapes
apple	blackberries
fresh dates	melon
orange	mango
pear	passion fruit
pineapple	cherries
peach	raspberries

1 Pour the fruit juice into a serving dish.
2 Peel, core and prepare the fruit and cut into even-sized pieces.
3 Add to the fruit juice, mix well and chill before serving.

Tropical Fruit Salad

Serves 4

A delicious dessert can be made for entertaining by making a fruit salad of tropical fruits, such as sharon fruit, dates, bananas, and mango, and mixing with 425ml/¾ pint/2 cups of yogurt (preferably Greek) instead of the fruit juice. Add ½ cup of toasted flaked almonds and assemble just before serving to prevent the yogurt becoming watery and the nuts soft.

Fruit Terrine

Serves 4

Gelozone is the vegetarian equivalent of gelatine. Use fruit juice from a carton rather than freshly squeezed as this is slightly less acidic. Other fruits can be substituted, such as pear, peach, sharon fruit, bananas and strawberries.

115g/4 oz/⅔ cup cherries	5ml/1 tsp Gelozone
115g/4 oz/¾ cup grapes	285ml/10 fl oz/1⅓ cups fruit
1 mango	juice
¼ melon	

1 Peel and stone the fruit and dice the mango and melon. Layer the fruit in a terrine or loaf tin.
2 Mix the Gelozone with the fruit juice in a pan and stir until dissolved.
3 Bring just to the boil then pour over the fruit in the terrine while still hot.
4 Refrigerate until set, then serve cut into slices.

Fruit Platter

The same ingredients can be used as for the previous recipe but served on individual plates (preferably white). Pour the fruit juice and Gelozone onto plates and arrange the fruit in an attractive pattern in the middle. Allow to set as before.

Jelly

A plain jelly can be made for children by using 570ml/1 pint/2½ cups of fruit juice and 10ml/1 level dsp Gelozone. Dissolve the Gelozone in the fruit juice in a pan then bring to the boil, stirring all the time. Place in a serving dish or mould and allow to cool in the fridge. Serve with fresh fruit, ice cream, yogurt or custard.

Banana and Mango Ice Cream

Serve the ice cream just as it is or with other puddings. Vary by adding toasted nuts, desiccated coconut or 15ml/1 tbsp carob flour. Finely chopped crystallized ginger or candied peel can be added for those allowed a little sugar, or for a dessert when entertaining.

3 bananas	140ml/5 fl oz/⅔ cup soya, rice
1 large mango	*or* almond milk

1 Peel and slice the bananas and freeze in a container so that the bananas are not squashed together but will separate when frozen.
2 Peel and stone the mango and dice the flesh. Freeze in the same way as the bananas.
3 Pour the milk into a food processor and switch on at full power. I wrap a tea towel round the processor to stop the milk splashing. Gradually add the banana and mango pieces through the funnel, stopping if necessary to break the fruit up if it starts to stick together. Eventually you will obtain a smooth, creamy ice cream.
4 Serve at once or return to the freezer. If left in the freezer for long, the ice cream will set quite hard and will then need to be left out to stand for approximately 20 minutes before serving.

Banana and Peace Ice Cream

Substitute 2 peaches for the mango in the previous recipe.

Strawberry and Banana Ice Cream

Substitute 285ml/10 oz/2 cups strawberries for the mango in the recipe for Banana and Mango Ice Cream *(see above)*. Allow the strawberries to thaw for approximately 5 minutes before processing as they are very solid when frozen.

Strawberry and Peach Sorbet

Freeze 285ml/10 oz/2 cups strawberries and 2 peaches. Thaw for approximately 5 minutes then process along with 115ml/4 fl oz/½ cup fruit juice (orange, apple etc.) or water.

A wide range of ice creams and sorbets can be made using the above methods and substituting different fruits. Yogurt can be used instead of the milk for another variation.

Sweet Soufflé Omelette

Serves 2

Mincemeat *(see Chapter 9, page 230)* or Marmalade *(see Chapter 1, page 60)* could be used instead of stewed fruit to fill the soufflé omelette.

2 eggs	90ml/6 tbsp stewed fresh fruit
30ml/2 tbsp water	e.g. apples, plums, apricots,
5ml/1 tsp sunflower oil	raspberries, blackberries,
	strawberries

1 Separate the egg yolks from the whites, putting them in two bowls. Add the water to the yolks and mix well.
2 Whisk the egg whites until stiff and fold gently into the egg yolks with a metal spoon.
3 Cook in the sunflower oil in an omelette pan over a medium heat until the underside of the omelette is golden brown.
4 Place the pan under the grill until the omelette is brown on top and set.
5 Spread the stewed fruit over the omelette and fold in half. Serve at once.

Stuffed Pancakes

Serves 4

1 egg	170ml/6 fl oz/¾ cup soya *or* rice milk
115g/4 oz/⅔ cup rice flour	60ml/2 fl oz/¼ cup water
3ml/½ tsp cinnamon	5ml/1 tsp baking powder
2ml/¼ tsp lemon rind	10ml/1 dsp sunflower oil

1 Blend all the ingredients except the oil in the food processor. If mixing by hand, beat the eggs then add the remaining ingredients except the oil and beat well.
2 Oil a pan or griddle and cook 4 pancakes. Turn the pancakes as soon as they are puffed and full of bubbles.

Banana Pancakes

Roll each pancake round a small peeled banana. Heat through and serve with soya yogurt, Banana and Mango Ice Cream *(see page 251)*, Carob Cream *(see page 236)* or Vanilla Custard *(see page 244)*.

Summer Fruit Pancakes

Gently stew a selection of summer fruits, such as strawberries, raspberries, redcurrants and blackberries. The juice could be thickened with a little arrowroot or Gelozone if desired. Serve layered with the pancakes.

Orange Pancakes

Fold the pancakes into quarters and warm in the pan with 140ml/¼ pint/⅔ cup of orange juice, the grated rind of ½ an orange and a few orange segments.

Apple Pancakes

Serve the pancakes with stewed apple sprinkled with nutmeg and cinnamon. Accompany with Vanilla Custard *(see page 244)* or Mango and Banana Ice Cream *(see page 251)* if desired.

Melon with Mango Sauce

Serves 4

1 small *or* ½ large melon	3 passion fruit
1 large *or* 2 small mangoes	

1 Cube or ball the melon flesh. Peel the mango and slice the flesh from the stone.
2 Liquidize the mango, the flesh from the passion fruit and a quarter of the melon to make a smooth sauce. If you have used a melon baller for the melon, liquidize the leftover pieces of melon.
3 Sieve the sauce to remove the passion fruit seeds. Serve the melon in sundae glasses with the sauce poured over.

Spiced Pears

Serves 4

The pears can be served hot or cold accompanied, if desired, with Vanilla Custard (see page 244), soya yogurt or Banana and Mango Ice Cream *(see page 251)*.

3 large firm pears	2ml/¼ tsp ground cloves
3ml/½ tsp ground cardamom	115ml/4 fl oz/½ cup apple juice
3ml/½ tsp cinnamon	

1 Peel and quarter the pears and cut away the cores.
2 Cut the pears into 2-cm/½-inch lengthwise slices and place in an ovenproof dish.
3 Sprinkle with the spices and pour the apple juice over.
4 Cover and bake at 400°F/200°C/Gas Mark 6 for approximately 20 minutes or until tender.

Poached Pears with Carob Custard

Serves 4

Serve hot or cold.

2 large pears	710ml/1¼ pints/3¼ cups soya *or*
45ml/3 tbsp water	almond milk
80ml/4 rounded tbsp rice flour	30ml/2 tbsp desiccated coconut
30ml/2 level tbsp carob flour	to decorate

1 Peel, core and quarter the pears and simmer gently in the water until just cooked.
2 Mix the rice flour and the carob flour with a little cold milk in a pan until smooth. Add the remaining milk and bring to the boil, stirring all the time. Simmer for 1 minute.
3 Serve the pears with the carob custard and sprinkled with the coconut.

Christmas Pudding

Makes 3 puddings to serve 4 people

I freeze any puddings which will not be used within one week as they will not keep for too long. Serve with vanilla custard.

1 portion of Christmas Cake recipe *(see page 228)*	225g/8 oz/2 cups baking apples, peeled and grated
2 large carrots, grated	20ml/2 level dsp baking powder

1 Mix the Christmas Cake ingredients as per the recipe on page 228. (To save time, I double the quantity and make both puddings and cake on the same day.)
2 Mix in the grated carrots, apples and baking powder.
3 Divide the mixture into greased pudding basins, depending on the size of the puddings you require.
4 Steam, pressure cook or microwave the puddings according to their size. The 4-person pudding will take 30 minutes in the pressure cooker, 2 hours over boiling water and 12 minutes in the microwave on power level 5.

List of Suppliers

Global Nutritional Products Ltd
48 Margarite Road, Tiverton, Devon, EX16 6TD
Tel and Fax 01884 251777
Suppliers of potassium baking powder and nutritional supplements.

Gordons Fine Foods
Gordon House, Littlemead, Cranleigh, Surrey, GU6 8ND
Tel 01483 267707 Fax 01483 267783
Mail order suppliers of mustard flour with no added ingredients and
    English mustard with salt, water and spices added.

Rio Trading Co (Health) Ltd
2 Centenary Estate, Hughes Rd, Brighton, East Sussex, BN2 4AW
Tel 01273 570987 Fax 01273 691226
Mail order suppliers of Stevia herbal sugar alternative.

Hambledon Herbs
Court Farm, Milverton, Somerset, TA4 1NF
Tel 01823 401205 Fax 01823 400276
Mail order suppliers of organic herbs and spices.

Neals Yard
29 John Dalton Street, Manchester, M2 6DS
Tel 0161 831 7875 Fax 0161 835 9322
Mail order suppliers of herbs and spices.

Swinton Health Foods
177 Moorside Road, Swinton, Manchester, M27 9LD
Tel 0161 793 0091 Fax 0161 793 0091
Mail order suppliers of alternative and substitute foods, books and
    nutritional supplements.

Useful Addresses

SPNT (Society for the Promotion of Nutritional Therapy)
PO Box 85, St Albans, Herts, AL3 7ZQ
An educational and campaigning organisation with lay and practitioner
  members. Send SAE and £1 for information and a list of your
  nearest qualified nutritional therapists.

ION (The Institute of Optimum Nutrition)
Blades Court, Deodar Road, London, SW15 2NU
Tel 0181 877 9993 Fax 0181 877 9980
ION exists as an independent charity to help you achieve optimum
  health. ION offers short courses, home study courses, books, a
  magazine, consultations and a Nutrition Consultants diploma
  course.

Higher Nature Ltd
Burwash Common, East Sussex, TN19 7LX
Tel 01435 882880 Fax 01435 883720
Catologue of nutritional supplements and free magazine available on
  request. Also nutritional helpline for your queries, or nutrition
  consultations by phone, or in person.

The Nutritional Cancer Therapy Trust
Skyecroft, Wonham Way, Gomshall, Surrey, GU5 9NZ
Tel 01483 202264 Fax 01483 203130
A registered charity assisting in the application of natural therapies for
  the remission of cancer and other degenerative diseases.

York Nutritional Laboratory
Murton Way, Osbaldwick, York, Y19 5US
Tel 01904 410410 Fax 01904 422000
Provides 'pin prick' blood testing for allergies and food sensitivities to
the general public, doctors and practitioners.

Allergy Care
1 Church Square, Taunton, Somerset, TA1 1SA
Tel 01823 325023 Fax 01823 325024
Mail order suppliers of some alternative and substitute food products.
Also a team of qualified allergy testers (using vega testing) working
in over 700 centres throughout the UK.

Alan Hopewell
South Gables, 2 Eleanor Rd, Bidston, Wirral, CH43 7QR
Tel 0151 652 4277 Fax 0161 652 5477
A bio-resonance practitioner who heads a group of holistic therapists
throughout the United Kingdom who offer allergy testing (using
vega testing) and nutritional advice.

Further Reading

Philosophy of Natural Therapeutics by Henry Lindlahr MD
CW Daniel Co. 1975. ISBN 0 85207 155 8

Hypoglycemia, a better approach by Dr Paavo Airola
Health Plus. 1997. ISBN 0 932090 01 X

Fats that Heal, Fats that Kill by Udo Erasmus
Alive Books. 1987. ISBN 0 920470 38 6

Candida Albicans by Leon Chaitow
Thorsons. 1996. ISBN 0 7225 3343 8

Healing with Whole Foods (oriental traditions and modern nutrition) by
    Paul Pitchford
North Atlantic Books. 1993. ISBN 0 938190 64 4

Nine Ways to Body Wisdom by Jennifer Harper
Thorsons. 1999. ISBN 0 7225 3368 3k

The Healing Power of Illness by Thorwald Dethlefsen
Element. 1999. ISBN 186 204 080 X

Heal Thyself by Dr Edward Bach
The CW Daniel Co. 1995. ISBN 0 85207 301 1

You Can Heal Your Life by Louise Hay
Eden Grove Editions. 1998. ISBN 1 870845 01 3

Bach Flower Therapy, The Complete Approach by Mechthild Scheffer.
Thorsons. 1990. ISBN 0 7225 1121 3

Index